Praise for *Solving the Anxiety Equation*

"As are many self-help books, *Solving the Anxiety Equation* is largely interactive, and includes helpful reflective, breathing, and writing exercises. But Ms. Leeds' illustrative personal narratives, so honest and self-revealing, and so well-written, greatly enrich this book. In fact, this is a bit of a page-turner and not easy to put down. With great empathy, she provides a cognitive but conversational explanation of self-doubt, the Fear of change, and physical anxiety, and then offers guidance for healing. Chapter titles like 'How to Handle Catastrophic Change' and subtitles such as 'This Is the Most Important Thing I've Ever Learned about Getting through a Tough Time' exemplify the author's willingness to share, directly and unabashedly, her own experience with anxiety. The reader becomes the confidante while remaining the focus of the endeavor; this encourages the reader to trust the psychotherapist and her process. This is skillfully accomplished and the result is one of the best self-help books this reviewer has read."

—**Roberta Rosenthal Hawkins, PhD**

"Unpack your anxiety and banish it forever with this honest and actionable recovery strategy. *Solving the Anxiety Equation* is a fully personalized plan to help you overcome the debilitating fears that prevent you from living a full and happy life. Part workbook and part advice manual, it takes readers on a journey to discover how their own form of anxiety shapes their world and what steps they can take to overcome it. This book does a phenomenal job of unpacking the different types of anxieties that inflict us and how to address each of them. This book is a rare breed—excellent for beginners and for those who have been struggling to overcome their anxieties for some time. You won't regret taking a chance on this one."

—**Joelene Pynnonen,** *Independent Book Review*

"A must-read for anyone who lives with anxiety. Wendy Leeds combines her personal experience as an anxious person, her work as a psychotherapist, her knowledge of research studies, and her exceptional writing skills to create a book that is easy to read, informative, and inspiring! As someone who has tried to manage anxiety my whole life, I found this book to be validating. As I read it, I felt understood and empowered. The book helps you understand the underlying causes of anxiety and then supplies the reader with many ways to overcome it. As Wendy says in this powerful book, we 'Don't have to settle.'"

—**Lucille R. Fisher**

"A conversational yet authoritative guide on navigating stress, strife, fear, and doubt, *Solving the Anxiety Equation: The Formula to Free Yourself from Fear* by Wendy Leeds is a timely companion for the increasingly worried masses. Probing into the fundamental aspects of anxiety and exemplifying these concepts with anecdotal stories and the author's own lived experience, this book offers an interactive self-assessment, which gradually leads the reader toward a tailored plan for stress reduction. Given the epidemic of anxiety and depression currently affecting people of all ages, Leeds' invaluably personalized take provides an accessible, compassionate, and customizable approach to reclaiming personal peace in a world that seems to be growing more chaotic."

—*Self-Publishing Review*

"*Solving the Anxiety Equation* is a compassionate and comprehensive guide to understanding and overcoming anxiety. It is an essential read for anyone looking to reclaim their life from the clutches of fear, providing hope and practical solutions that promise to empower readers. It's also beneficial for those living with someone suffering from anxiety to understand better what the person is experiencing. Leeds provides a plethora of references for further reading and it's a book to refer to often."

—**Carol Thompson**, *Readers' Favorite*

"Wendy Leeds masterfully tells the story of anxiety, both from a personal perspective and a professional one. This book offers a clear definition of anxiety, followed by a journey through its root causes, culminating with an array of techniques for managing and mastering it. There is something for everyone who suffers from anxiety in the book."

—**Peg Doyle, MEd**

Solving the Anxiety Equation

Solving THE Anxiety Equation

The Formula to
Free Yourself
from Fear

WENDY LEEDS

Solving the Anxiety Equation: The Formula for Freeing Yourself from Fear
© 2024 Wendy Leeds

All rights reserved. No part of this publication may be reproduced in any form or by any electronic or mechanical means, including information storage and retrieval systems, without permission in writing by the publisher, except by a reviewer who may quote brief passages in a review. For information regarding permission, contact the publisher at calmdaypublishing@gmail.com.

Published by Calm Day Publishing
wendyleeds.com
Medfield, MA

Paperback ISBN: 978-0-9999015-4-0
Ebook ISBN: 978-0-9999015-5-7

Cover and interior design by Liz Schreiter
Illustrations by Thomas Leeds
Edited and produced by Reading List Editorial
ReadingListEditorial.com

This book is dedicated to my mom,
Shirley M. Buck.
Thanks for leading the way.

Contents

Welcome 1

Part One:
Getting Started

1: Are You Anxious? 11
2: What's Making Us Anxious? 14
3: The Anxiety Equation 19

Part Two:
Self-Doubt

4: What Is Self-Doubt? 24
5: What Causes Self-Doubt? 27
6: Start Telling Your Story Differently 33
7: So, Who Do You Think You Are? 35
8: Who You Really Are 38
9: Talk about Your Story Differently 44
10: Five Simple Phrases That Can Change Your Life 46
11: Letting Go of the Story of Your Past 51
12: Forgiving 54
13: Our Story about the Future 59
14: Act as If 64
15: Telling the Hero's Story 68

Part Three:
The Fear of Change

16: What Is the Fear of Change? 73
17: What Causes the Fear of Change? 76
18: Giving Up the Need to Be in Charge of the Universe 80
19: Thought Swapping 84

20: What Do You Really Want? 88
21: How to Get What You Really Want 92
22: Travel Light: Clearing Out the Clutter 97
23: Birds That Flock Together: The Power of Our Relationships . . 104
24: How to Handle Catastrophic Change 109
25: The BEAR Technique to Stop or Prevent Panic Attacks 112

Part Four:
Physical Anxiety

26: What Is Physical Anxiety? 117
27: It's the Vagus, Baby 121
28: What Causes Physical Anxiety? 127
29: The Price We Pay for Physical Anxiety 131
30: Just Breathe 134
31: Meditation 140
32: Acupressure 146
33: Massage 154
34: A Body in Motion 157
35: Splash Some Cold Water on It 161
36: Music 164
37: Laughter 166

Part Five:
Creating Your Personalized Plan for Healing Your Anxiety

38: Find Out What's Really Causing Your Anxiety: The Quiz 171
39: Getting Started 175
40: Staying on Track 179

Conclusion: The Journey Ahead 183
References 184
Acknowledgments 191
About Wendy Leeds 192

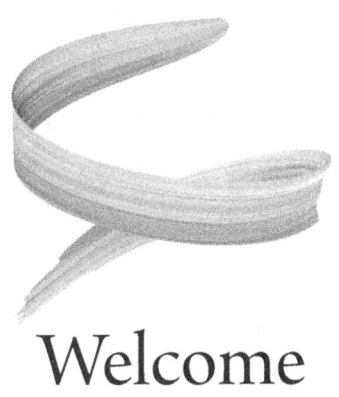

Welcome

If you've picked up this book, I'm betting we're a lot alike. I bet you're anxious like me. I bet you've struggled with your anxiety the way I have. I bet you're tired of living in fear. I bet you've tried some ways to feel better but haven't found what works for you. And I bet you're ready to move past that fear and into the life you were born to live.

Me too!

Let Me Introduce Myself

First of all, I'm a world-class expert on anxiety. I'm not only a licensed psychotherapist with an interest in anxiety, but I've also been anxious for as long as I can remember.

I grew up in an anxious family. We worried about everything. My father actually made lists of things to worry about from the smallest to the largest. You name it, we worried about it.

And I thought everyone else worried the same way we did. I thought my classmates were terrified that they'd be called on in class. I thought they stayed awake nights worrying about having to take a test or sit alone in the cafeteria. And as I got older, I thought my friends felt nauseous before a social event or spent time imagining how their plane was going to crash or how they were going to end up homeless.

And while I believed we all thought the same way about the world, I noticed it didn't seem to bother everyone else the way it bothered me.

And I decided that everyone else was in on a secret that I just didn't get. They were somehow better than me. I thought there was something wrong with me.

So, I worried my way all through school and on into adulthood. And I probably would have just kept on worrying if it weren't for the moment that changed my life.

Aha!

Years ago, I remember telling my husband how worried I was about the upcoming holidays. I remember telling him how concerned I was that we weren't going to be able to get the house clean and the shopping and the cooking done in time. He was listening but didn't seem concerned. And I remember saying to him, "Aren't you worried?"

He looked at me and shrugged. "What's there to worry about?"

I remember being stunned and silent for a moment. Was he kidding? What's there to be worried about? Everything! And I started reading him the to-do list.

"What if the house isn't clean? What if the food isn't great? What if we give someone the wrong present? What if we don't get all the decorations up or get the baking done in time?"

"So what?" he said.

"So *what*?" What was wrong with him? Couldn't he see how important it was to make sure we got everything done on time and without mistakes? Why wasn't he worried about what people would think and say about us if we failed? Why wasn't he panicked and overwhelmed at the thought of things not being perfect?

When I was done reading the list, he shrugged and said what he always says: "It'll be all right."

"No, it won't," I said right back, thinking there was something really wrong with him because he couldn't see how stressful and terrifying the whole thing was.

He looked more confused than ever. "How do you know?"

"I know because . . ." I started, and then I stopped because I realized I *didn't* know. Neither of us knew what was going to happen. But he was choosing to believe things would work out and was able to go on with his life.

I, on the other hand, was imagining the worst. I was paralyzing myself with fearful thoughts about things that possibly might happen in the future. I was thinking thoughts that were making me miserable—and they were all made up. *None of them were true.*

I remember standing there thinking, "What if this isn't about him? What if it's about *me*?"

And that was the moment I realized that all my worrying wasn't normal. I had anxiety.

I remember being both shocked and relieved. Shocked at the idea that there were people who didn't worry all the time. And relieved I finally had a name for what was causing me so much pain and misery. It was a big step forward, but it didn't give me a clue about how to feel better.

So, I continued to suffer in silence. And I kept telling myself I was doing okay—until the day the doctor called to tell me I had breast cancer. That changed everything.

A Cancer Diagnosis Changes Everything

I thought I knew what it was like to be afraid, but after that diagnosis, the next six months of surgery and chemo were beyond endurance. It wasn't the physical pain of the treatment that was so tough to bear; it was the fear. Both my days and my nights were haunted by thoughts of despair, illness, loss, grief, and death. And I suffered the fear in silence. After all, good people don't burden anyone else with their fear. And sharing those fears would make me look weak and helpless, and everyone would see that there was something wrong with me. They would realize what I already knew: I wasn't good enough.

To be honest, at one point I reached a place so deep and dark I couldn't see a way out.

And not long after that a miracle happened for me.

Read All about It

Someone gave me a book on anxiety. I heard Tony Robbins and Louise Hay speak, and I bought their books. And then I discovered the work of Joan Borysenko, Aaron Beck, Martha Beck, and so many other amazing writers who understood what I was going through. And I realized that the library and bookstores were full of books on how to face our fears.

I wasn't the only one who was afraid! There were lots of people who thought the way I did, and some of them had found ways to deal with that fear. Wow!

I started trying some of those suggestions in my own life. Some worked, some didn't. But I kept with it, and over time I was able to put together an entire tool kit of simple things I could do to help me feel better in the moment and to create an ongoing sense of calm in my life.

It's Not Just Me

I went back to graduate school to study counseling psychology, and I continued to learn everything I could about anxiety. Eventually I started to share what I was learning with clients, then friends, family, and anyone else who'd listen. "We don't have to suffer anymore," I'd tell them. "There are things we can do to feel better." I found that everyone's anxiety looked a little different. Not every technique worked for everyone, but we could always come up with something that helped.

I loved sharing what I knew. I loved working with clients and helping them feel better. And I thought at last I had my happy, anxiety-free ending. It turns out I was wrong!

Cancer Again

Fifteen years after my original diagnosis of breast cancer, my doctor called to tell me that I had leukemia.

Cancer again.

Once again, I faced that hot, sweaty fear of the unknown. I faced chemo and long months of recovery, and, I have to admit, I was scared. But it was different this time. This time I didn't experience the crippling fear I'd experienced fifteen years earlier. This time I knew I had solutions, I had answers. I had all sorts of ways to ease my fears and bring peace to my body and mind. This time was different because *I* was different.

And Again

I made it through that treatment and spent years in remission. And then my doctor called to tell me that I had leukemia again.

Boy, I wish I could tell you that I breezed my way through chemo this third time. But it was still a tough battle. I still had moments of terrible fear, I still felt panicky and suffered some sleepless nights. But this time, though I still got anxious, I no longer had to stay anxious.

And today I'm proud to say that I'm a three-time cancer survivor.

What about You?

I'm sitting down to write this book so I can share all the things I've learned over the years in my journey to find peace in my own life. Because I know I'm not the only one suffering in silence.

I can't tell you how many times I've shared the story of my anxiety with people who nod in agreement. I hear replies like "Oh, me too," or "My sister won't get on an airplane," or "My child is afraid to go to school," or "My whole family is anxious. But we're not allowed to talk about it."

So, let me ask you: What's your story? Maybe it's something like mine. Maybe anxiety runs in your family. Or maybe you've experienced a difficult life event or a life-changing trauma—or more than one trauma—that triggered fear and panic in you.

Maybe you're afraid to drive, to fly, or to go to medical appointments. Maybe you're afraid to leave your house. Maybe you're afraid to go back home.

Fear comes in all sorts of forms and sizes. It shows up differently for all of us. It can be predictable, or it can show up unexpectedly.

But no matter how it shows up, anxiety can make us sick physically. It can limit our lives, keep us from succeeding at work or school. It can drain the love and joy out of our relationships, and it can make us doubt or even hate ourselves.

Anxiety can make us ashamed of ourselves, of who we are and what we can do. And so maybe you're working hard to hide your fears. Maybe, like I was, you're suffering in silence. Maybe you're telling yourself that things are all right when you know they're not. Maybe you believe that having anxiety means you're weak, broken, or not good enough.

But let's start off this journey together by acknowledging that none of those negative thoughts are true!

The Truth about Our Anxiety

I'm not broken, and neither are you.

Anxious people like us aren't weak. In fact, we're the exact opposite. We're stronger and more courageous than the people around us. We have to be because it's twice as hard to get out of bed in the morning when you're full of fear. It takes courage and strength to make it through our days.

More importantly, anxiety doesn't just happen to us. Anxiety is learned and can be unlearned. I promise you there are all sorts of things

Welcome

we can do to feel better right now and for the rest of our lives. And thanks to the *anxiety equation*, it's easier than you might think.

Part One

Getting Started

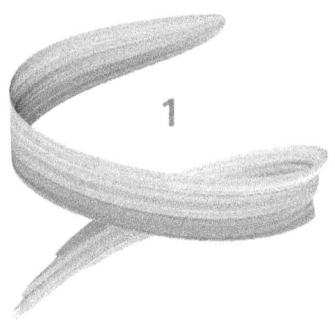

Are You Anxious?

Do you worry about your worrying?
Everyone worries from time to time. In fact, worry is a normal reaction to much of what happens to us in life. But while everyone worries, not everyone has anxiety.

What's the difference?

The Birds of Worry

The simplest way I can explain the difference between worry and anxiety is this old Chinese proverb: "The birds of worry and care fly over your head, this you cannot change, but that they build nests in your hair, this you can prevent."

Exactly!

Worry

Worry is that bird that flies over our heads and then soars back into the sky. Worry is our normal response to life. It's short term, and it's usually in response to a specific situation. While it can be annoying or unpleasant, you can usually control your worry. Worry doesn't have a long-term negative impact on your life; in fact, it can help keep you safe. Worry makes sure we have a fire extinguisher in our kitchen and we go to the dentist when our tooth hurts.

On the other hand, anxiety is that bird that nests in our hair and makes us miserable.

Anxiety

Unlike worry, anxiety isn't normal. And unlike worry, which usually happens in your head, anxiety can cause physical symptoms like a rapid heartbeat, headaches, digestive complaints, chills, shaking, sweating, and insomnia. Worry is usually sparked by some real difficulty, like paying taxes or getting your car fixed. Anxiety tends to be more generalized and is usually the product of our overactive imagination.

But the most important difference between worry and anxiety is the impact each has on our life. While worry flies overhead every now and again, anxiety really does come and nest in our hair.

And it can seriously alter our life. Anxiety can affect our job performance, our relationships, and our physical health. It can feel so overwhelming that we think we're not able to handle it.

Worst of all, anxiety can make us feel out of control and hopeless.

So, What about You?

Are you a worrier? Or, like me, are you dealing with anxiety?

If you're not sure, take this true/false quiz.

Worry vs. Anxiety Quiz

- T - F: I worry about everything.
- T - F: I worry all the time.
- T - F: Worry keeps me from doing things I need or want to do.
- T - F: Worry keeps me awake.

T - F: I have unexplained physical symptoms, like digestive issues, headaches, numbness, tingling, shortness of breath, exhaustion, or insomnia.

T - F: I worry about things that aren't real. They're just things I imagine *might* happen.

T - F: I feel like I can't control my worry.

T - F: My worry isn't short term. It's ongoing.

T - F: My worry is impacting my relationships, my career, and/or my health.

T - F: My worry gets in the way of living my best life.

If you answered true to three or more of these questions, chances are that your anxiety is keeping you from living the life you really want.

If you're a worrier, feel free to stick around. We're glad you're here. But if you're anxious (or you know someone who is), let's take a closer look at your anxiety and figure out the best way for you to get started easing those fears.

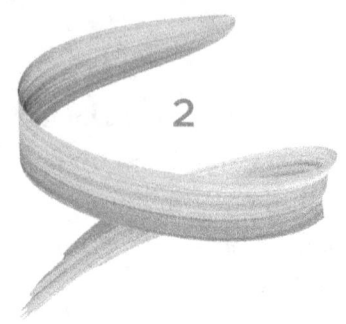

What's Making Us Anxious?

Let's begin at the beginning—by defining anxiety. I define anxiety as the fear that you won't be able to handle things that *might* happen to you in the future. It's your response to the fear and trauma of the past, which causes you to doubt yourself and results in physical tension.

And in that definition are all three causes of our anxiety. Anxiety is caused by our fearful thoughts about the future, the trauma and failures from our past, and physical stress with its unpleasant and sometimes debilitating symptoms.

It sounds complicated, but let's break it down and look at these causes one by one.

The Past

Our past plays a major role in our anxiety. And I'm not just talking about our *personal* past but the whole history of humankind as well.

Our Collective Past

According to evolutionary psychology, the brains of our earliest ancestors were wired to focus on the negative to keep them alive. Focusing on fearful thoughts about possible future dangers helped them prepare for the worst.[1]

Worrying about running out of food, having enough firewood, or whether a lion could be lurking somewhere close by meant they were able to store food, stockpile firewood, and create a tool to defend themselves from animal attacks.

And today our brains are wired the same way. As Rick Hanson, PhD, psychologist and *New York Times* best-selling author, writes, "The brain is like Velcro for negative experiences but Teflon for positive ones."[2] Exactly!

But the dangers we face today are not so alarming or life threatening. Today we worry about things like being stuck in traffic, being overdrawn at the bank, or our boss's bad moods—things we have no control over, things that tend to be chronic. And all that long-term worrying can do considerable ongoing harm to our brains and our bodies.

But that's not the only part of our past that can make us anxious.

Our Personal Past

The trauma and drama of our *personal* past can also play a major role in making us anxious. As Donald O. Hebb suggests in his influential 1949 book, *The Organization of Behavior*, "Neurons that fire together, wire together."[3] In other words, we're most likely to remember events and incidents that evoke an intense emotional reaction in us.

While we struggle to remember what we had for breakfast on Tuesday, we're likely to remember every detail of the shame we felt when our fifth-grade teacher announced to the class that we couldn't spell. We remember the horror and embarrassment of not being prepared in that meeting, or the terror of crashing head on into the guardrail.

And we often remember that fear, pain, or shame in great detail. All those failures and disasters get stored away in our brains in Technicolor, just waiting to be triggered by a story: frightening evening news, a nasty comment by your partner, or the rumble of thunder.

And the more we revisit those vivid, traumatic memories, the more likely they are to become a part of who and what we believe we are in the present.

Over time those negative memories can cause us to doubt ourselves. They can lead us to believe that we're not capable, all we do is fail, and we're not good enough.

It's those old stories we repeat to ourselves that cause our self-doubt. And that self-doubt is what makes us so afraid of what's ahead of us.

If we can't handle the past, how the heck are we going to be able to handle the future?

The Future

Our thoughts about what's in our future can make us really anxious, but maybe not in the way you think. *At least not the way I used to think about it.*

Rethinking Our Thinking

I'd always thought my anxiety was a reaction to life around me—my internal response to an external event.

For instance, "I'm afraid of snakes, so it must be those snakes that make me anxious."

But I've realized that for the most part, anxiety isn't a matter of snakes, the fear of public speaking, or the worry about losing your job—anxiety is actually about what you think and feel before you see the snake, have to speak, or meet with your boss.

It's what I call a *preaction*, or an action that happens *before* the thing that might or might not happen. Just the way a reaction happens after something takes place, a preaction happens before.

I don't even need to see a snake to be anxious. Just thinking about seeing a snake makes me anxious. Actually, seeing that snake wouldn't make me anxious; it would make me terrified, and I would probably freeze in place with fear!

So, for the most part, anxiety happens *before* events or challenges that may or may not take place.

Here's what I'm talking about.

Preaction →	Event →	Reaction
Our thoughts and concerns about what might happen. The negative things we tell ourselves make us anxious.	The event happens or does not happen	Our actions in response to the event

We don't worry after something's happened because we know how it turned out.

Anxiety is caused by the thinking we do *before* the thing happens. It's those negative stories we make up. It's the product of our imagination, and it can make us miserable.

So, anxiety is caused by the trauma from our past plus our fear of the future. But there's one more important cause of our anxiety I haven't mentioned yet, and it's one that only occurs in the present: physical anxiety.

The Present

Recent research has shown that anxiety isn't just in our heads. Our bodies can actually make our brains anxious. We've known for a long time that our bodies and our minds are connected and that what we *feel* can have a real effect on our body. But now we know that works the other way around as well. What our body feels can affect what we think.[4]

We now know that our body and brain are in constant communication through the vagus nerve. The signals between body and brain travel back and forth, and those signals from a tense, nervous body can cause a tense, anxious brain. In short, our bodies can make us anxious too. But we'll talk about that later.

The Moment of Power

While anxiety is caused by self-doubts from the past and worries about the future, we only experience our anxiety in the present. We can't change what happened in the past. We can't control what will happen in the future. But we *can* control how we show up in the present.

And that means the key to easing our anxiety always lies in this present moment, or what I call *the moment of power*.

Every new moment brings you the chance to begin again.

And why not claim this very moment as your moment of power? Right here and right now, you have the power to decide to move past your fear and take action to create the peaceful, calm life you've always dreamed of having.

And we're going to do that by using the anxiety equation.

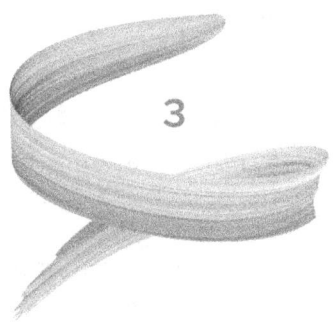

The Anxiety Equation

The anxiety equation isn't about numbers. It's a way of describing anxiety that's clear, concise, and easy to understand at a glance.

The anxiety equation breaks anxiety down into its three parts so we can see exactly how each part works on its own—and then how those parts function together to create our worries and fears.

Curious?

Well, here's the equation.

Anxiety = Self-Doubt + Fear of Change + Physical Anxiety

Now, this may look like just a simple equation. But don't let that simplicity fool you. This equation has the power to change your life. I know because it's changed mine.

So, let's take a look at how we can use the anxiety equation to solve our own anxiety in three easy steps.

Here's how it works:

Step 1: We take the mystery out of anxiety.
We'll begin by looking at each of the three factors of the equation in depth.

- First, we'll explore the causes and impact of self-doubt, and we'll examine our beliefs about whether we can handle what life throws at us.
- Next, we'll talk about the scary stories we tell ourselves about what may or may not happen in the future. We'll look at how those stories can make us afraid of change.
- Finally, we'll examine the sources of physical anxiety and its impact on our lives.

Once we have a clear understanding of how each of these factors work, we're going to explore the most effective way to heal each one.

When we use the anxiety equation, we don't have to guess where our anxiety comes from or wonder how it's making our lives so miserable. And we don't have to guess which tools and techniques are best for each factor. We know.

So, step 1 is where we learn that anxiety isn't something that happens to us. It's something we can understand and control. Step 1 is about putting us in charge of our anxiety rather than letting it run our lives.

Step 2: We take the mystery out of your anxiety.
No doubt about it, anxiety isn't the same for everyone. Over the years, I've heard all sorts of descriptions of what anxiety looks like, including the following:

"Anxiety is the voice of a relentless bully—judging, criticizing, and reminding me that I'm never going to be good enough, and I'm never going to do enough to be good enough."

"Anxiety makes me feel like I'm trapped in a fog of fear that keeps me trapped in a loop of negative thoughts."

"Anxiety makes me feel like I'm underwater and I can't breathe."

"Anxiety makes me feel like I always have to be ready to fight. I walk around with my body tense and my mind on full alert."

"Anxiety makes me shake and sweat."

"When I'm really anxious, I feel like I'm going to throw up."

"Having a panic attack feels like I'm having a heart attack."

Any of these sound familiar? Or does your anxiety show up with its own individual set of signs and symptoms?

The truth is that your anxiety is unique to you. While we may share some common symptoms and responses—and we certainly share similar feelings about the devastation anxiety can wreak—your anxiety has its own set of causes, challenges, and choices. What works for me may not work for you, and vice versa.

And that means we all have to find our own path to healing our anxiety. Which brings us to step 3.

Step 3: We work together to create a personal plan for healing your anxiety.

I've learned from personal experience that the best way to work through your fear and anxiety is to have a clear, inspiring, and workable plan in place. Having that plan can give you the confidence to take that first step. It can keep you on track and help you navigate the tough times.

All you have to do to create that plan is take the quiz in chapter 38 to get a look at exactly how anxiety is showing up in your life. Then you can use the Weekly Success Planner to create a plan for healing that's right for you.

That's all there is to it. No wishing or hoping or guessing. Just a clear path to feeling better and everything you need to get there.

So, let's roll up our sleeves and get to work.

Part Two

Self-Doubt

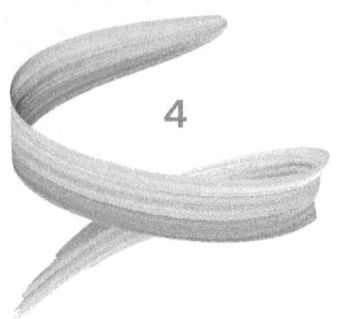

4

What Is Self-Doubt?

I learned to drive in a tan Dodge Dart. It had been my grandfather's car and was passed down to me. It was old. It was well used. And it was beige, inside and out.

It was a square, no-frills tank of a car. But it was perfect for someone learning to drive. And I really loved that car, in spite of its quirks. It had to be convinced to start on cold winter mornings. It shimmied a little if you went over fifty-five on the highway. And its emergency brake had a mind of its own. I mean that brake was crazy.

To put that emergency brake on, you had to step on a little emergency pedal that was to the far left of the brake pedal, over in the corner under the dashboard. And back in the day, you had to put on the emergency brake every time you parked if you didn't want your car to roll down the hill or drift across the parking lot and smash into something.

When I parked, I'd put on the brake by pressing that emergency brake pedal to the floor. And all would be well until I was ready to drive again. Then I'd have to release that brake. And that's when the trouble started.

To take off that emergency brake, I had to yank on the black handle underneath the dashboard to the left. But no matter how hard I pulled, I could never be sure whether or not those brakes were completely off.

The only way you could tell for sure was to put your foot on the gas and hope for the best.

If I'd fully released the brake, off I'd drive with no worries. But more often than not, the brakes were still partly engaged. If that was the case, the car would start moving forward as if nothing was wrong—but if I tried to go over ten or fifteen miles an hour, the car would suddenly start jolting forward, hiccuping and complaining.

And, as I learned from a really expensive experience, if you continued to try and force the car to go faster, eventually smoke would come out from under the hood and the car would smell like something was burning—because it was.

This made getting where I wanted to go really tough. For years that brake pedal held me back.

Self-doubt is exactly like that brake.

Self-doubt—all those thoughts you have of failure and defeat and shame and guilt—is what's holding you back. In my experience, when self-doubt is running things, it's like driving through life with one foot on the gas pedal and the other foot on the brake.

Simply put, self-doubt is the deeply held belief that you can't do something. You can't finish. You can't achieve. You can't connect. You can't hold up your end of a relationship. You can't get a good job. You can't take care of yourself in the world. You can't trust yourself—because you believe you're not good enough.

And this self-doubt, this emergency brake, could also be playing a big part in your anxiety.

Let's find out.

How Does Self-Doubt Impact Your Life?

Almost all of us have some negative thoughts and self-doubts at times. But for some of us, these self-doubts are running our lives and making us anxious.

Here are some ways self-doubt can affect our lives. See how many apply to you.

Self-doubt can:

- make it hard for you to make decisions. You have to ask everyone else before you decide to take any action.
- cause procrastination. You put off starting things because you're afraid to fail.
- keep you stuck because you're afraid to make a change in your life.
- make it hard for you to finish things. The minute things go wrong with a project, you quit rather than produce something less than perfect.
- make you feel like an impostor. No matter how much you succeed, you feel broken or flawed inside. You worry that people will find out your shameful secret.
- cause you to downplay your accomplishments or successes. You don't feel that you deserve acknowledgment or credit for anything you've done.
- create the need to be perfect in everything you do. You recheck your work. You second-guess yourself. You hesitate to speak up in case your answer is wrong.
- cause you to avoid conflict and difficult conversations at all costs.
- make you struggle to please everyone. You want everyone to like you, so you have trouble setting boundaries or asking for what you want. You let people take advantage of you, or you end up doing without.
- make you feel trapped in a life that isn't working for you.

If some of these statements resonated with you, I hope you'll keep reading. Because together we're going to take a look at what we can do to replace that doubt with a sense of trust and self-confidence.

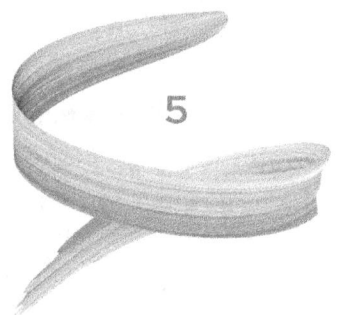

What Causes Self-Doubt?

There's no doubt about it: self-doubt is learned.

No one is born doubting themselves. Babies don't worry about whether or not they deserve to be fed. They demand food at the top of their lungs. They don't worry about the shape of their nose or the size of their belly. They love their bodies without judgment or criticism or doubt. They don't worry about whether or not people like them—they just expect it. And they love themselves.

We were all babies once. We all loved ourselves—once.

But most of us don't feel that way today. In fact, for most of us it's just the opposite. We spend our days judging ourselves harshly. We criticize what we think, how we feel, what we do, and how we look. We worry no one will like us. We remind ourselves over and over that we're not good enough. We tell ourselves we're somehow broken, and we worry someone else will find out what losers we really are.

So, what happened between then and now?

What We Learned in Childhood

One of the biggest factors influencing how we feel about ourselves is what we learned from our earliest caregivers. We learned a lot from what our parents or the people in authority told us about who we were, what we were capable of, and what we deserved. And those early lessons can play a powerful role in what we believe about ourselves today.

(And when I say *parents*, I'm not just talking about biological parents or caregivers. This can apply to any important adult figure who had an impact on your life.)

To give you a better idea of what I'm talking about, let's take a look at three little girls: Annie, Becky, and Carol. They're all the same age, but they have very different parents. As you read through these examples, see if anything sounds familiar. What kind of influence did your parents or caregivers have on your life?

Annie

Annie's parents are both really busy with work. They never have much time for Annie. One afternoon, Annie is playing on the front porch when she notices a big black spider on the other end of the porch. Annie yelps in fear and runs to tell her parents.

Her father says, "I'm busy. Leave me alone." Her mother says, "You're overreacting. There's nothing to be afraid of and for heaven's sake, stop interrupting when I'm working." Annie goes back to the porch to play as far away from the spider as possible. She is still afraid, and she is still alone. No one's going to help her.

So, what has Annie learned? She's learned that what she experiences and what she feels about it isn't valid or important. Her fears and needs are foolish. She's learned she can't trust her judgment. She's just a foolish, ineffectual little girl who needs to look outside herself for the answers rather than trust her own instincts.

Now, maybe this happens to Annie just once, but the event is so scary and memorable that it leaves a lasting impression. It becomes such a defining moment in her childhood that the idea she's not capable or worthy is wired in her brain.

Or maybe this kind of event happens over and over to Annie. And over time, when she realizes her efforts don't produce any results, she just gives up even asking for help. Maybe she begins to believe she's not worthy of being helped.

Becky

Becky's parents are angry most of the time either at her or each other, and they're always yelling. One afternoon, Becky is playing on the front porch when she sees a big black spider on the other end of the porch. Becky yelps in fear and runs to tell her parents. So, it's the same event, and Becky had the same reaction as Annie. But she gets a very different reaction from her parents.

Becky's mother shouts, "What is wrong with you! You need to stop whining and grow up." Her father yells, "I'll give you something to be really afraid of!"

Becky goes back to the porch and sits cowering in the corner. Alone. She now knows her needs, feelings, and thoughts are actually dangerous and can get her into some real trouble. She's also learned she's not okay. There's no question that there's something really wrong with her.

Carol

Carol's parents are both present for her and make her a priority in their lives. They aren't perfect, but they are there. One afternoon, Carol is playing on the front porch when she notices a big black spider. She yelps in fear and runs to her parents. Her mom puts an arm around Carol and her father gets rid of the spider.

Do you feel the difference? Carol's learned it's okay to ask for help. It's okay to be Carol.

You

So, think back to your childhood. What messages did you get from your parents, family, friends, or authority figures in your life? (As an aside, this is not about blaming anyone else. This is about you. It's about finding those places where you were hurt or given misinformation about your wonderful self. This is about looking to your past and using that information to help you move forward. No blame—just information.)

So, what about you? What messages did you get from the people around you when you were young?

Write them down here:

What were the positive messages? _____

_____

What were the negative messages? _____

_____

Can you identify some of the times when you learned not to trust or care for yourself? _____

_____

How does that impact your life today? _____

_____

Trauma

Years ago, my husband and I were driving back home after a lovely dinner out with a group of friends.

It was a bitterly cold winter night, and the road was narrow, icy, and dark.

As we went around a sharp turn, the car started to fishtail. I remember grabbing hold of the armrest and closing my eyes as the car spun fully around, then crashed headfirst into the cement barrier that divided the lanes.

We both sat there a moment in stunned silence. And then my husband asked, "Are you all right?"

"I'm okay," I said. "Are you okay?"

"I'm fine. Get out of the car," he ordered. "Now!"

And when I looked around, I realized that our car was sitting across the road, blocking oncoming traffic.

I remember climbing out of the car in the total darkness and going to the far side of the road. My husband grabbed a lantern and headed up the road, waving it to warn oncoming traffic. I remember yelling at him that he was going to get hit, and I recall the feeling of helplessness and loss of control. There was nothing I could do. I could only watch and worry.

The good news was that some wonderful people stopped to help us, and no one was hurt

The car was totaled, but we were both "okay." Or so I thought.

But it turned out I wasn't okay at all. I started having nightmares and trouble sleeping. And I was suddenly afraid to ride in a car with another driver. I avoided it when I could. And when I couldn't, I would sit in the passenger seat, heart pounding, gripping the armrest and pressing my right foot to the car floor as if I were pressing the brakes.

For me, the worst part of that car accident was that it left me feeling like I had no control of my life or myself. And that loss of control was terrifying.

What I didn't know then but can clearly see now is that I was suffering from trauma. And that trauma had a profound impact on my life.

It may be the same for you. Maybe you've experienced a trauma in your life that still haunts you. Maybe you've experienced more than one trauma. And maybe, like me, you experienced a trauma and didn't realize it.

Most of us think of trauma as a single catastrophic event: an accident, an assault, or an illness. But trauma can also be caused by long-term abuse—both physical and emotional.

Trauma can be caused by being shamed, bullied, mocked, ignored, or abandoned.

And it may surprise you to learn that you can experience trauma just by witnessing a traumatic event happening to someone else. Watching an accident, whether you're involved or not, can cause trauma. Even learning about a traumatic event that's happened to a close friend or family member can cause trauma.[5]

No matter what kind of trauma you've experienced, it can leave you feeling that life is dangerous and there's nothing you can do to keep yourself or those you love safe. It can convince you that you're not strong or smart or good enough to keep bad things from happening, no matter how hard you try.

And, as I've learned from personal experience, dealing with the aftermath of trauma can destroy our self-confidence and leave us feeling powerless and afraid. As Bessel van der Kolk, MD, writes in his book *The Body Keeps the Score*, "Trauma robs you of the feeling that you are in charge of yourself . . . The challenge of recovery is to establish ownership of your body and your mind—of yourself."[6]

And that's what we're going to do in the chapters ahead: recover and restore the ownership of you!

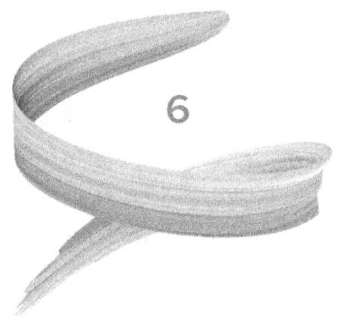

Start Telling Your Story Differently

As I've said, self-doubt is the inability to trust ourselves and our abilities. It's that judgy, unrelenting voice in our head reminding us 24/7 that we're not good enough—that we're broken, useless, and incompetent.

Self-doubt is a result of all that baggage we're all still dragging around with us, our history and all the trauma we've been through.

But it isn't the trauma itself that causes self-doubt—it's our reaction to that trauma. It's not the car accident; it's our fear about getting in that car again. It's not that your father called you stupid, or lazy, or a loser; it's how you've reacted to it. And it's how it made you feel about yourself, especially if you've chosen to repeat it to yourself so many times that you now believe it.

Self-doubt is an inside job.

Self-doubt doesn't happen *to* you. It happens *in* you!

The Story of Your Past

First of all, let's agree that it isn't fair that those terrible, unforgivable things happened to you. Those things weren't your fault. Yet here we are, putting the responsibility for your fear and self-doubt on your shoulders. But this is good news, actually: it means you don't have to depend on anyone or anything else to feel better. You don't have to wait for someone to come along and rescue you from the pain in your heart. You can do it yourself. All you have to do is start telling yourself the truth about what happened in your past and how you reacted to it.

Believe me, the stories we tell ourselves about our pasts matter. They define us, and they confine us to old beliefs, half truths, and other people's opinions. These stories tell us who we are in the world.

And while these stories are often made up of things other people have told you, the truth is this is *your* story. And that means you can change it, rewrite it, and edit it any way you want.

Now, I'm not talking about changing the facts. No one can change the past. But what you *can* change is what you tell yourself about how you handled the things that happened to you. And when you start telling yourself the truth about your past, and your strength and courage in facing some really hard times, you not only ease your anxiety in the present, but you lay the foundation for an amazing future.

So, Who Do You Think You Are?

To figure out who you really are, let's start by taking a quick look at what's happened to you over the years.

There are no rules here about how you should fill out this questionnaire. You can answer all the questions or none of them. You can answer just the one or two questions that really have meaning for you. You may have the same answer for one or more of the questions. You may begin to see a pattern or some connections that you hadn't noticed before.

Remember, there are no right or wrong answers—just the truth about what you've experienced in your life and how those events impacted you.

Write your name here: _____

Now, let's take a look at those life-changing moments.

1. The best moment of my life was _____

_____

Why? _____

2. The worst moment of my life was _____

_____

Why? _____

3. The scariest moment of my life was _____

_____

Why? _____

_____

4. The proudest moment of my life was _____

_____

Why? _____

5. My greatest success was _____

_____

Why? _____

6. My worst failure was _____

_____

Why? _____

7. The most peaceful time in my life was _____

_____

Why? _____

8. The angriest time in my life was _____

_____

Why? _____

9. The moment I felt the closest to another human being was _____

_____

Why? _____

10. The time I felt the loneliest was _____

_____

Why? _____

11. The deepest regret about my life is _____

_____

Why? _____

12. My deepest joy in my life is _____

_____

Why? _____

13. The theme(s) of my life is/are _____

_____

So, now that we've collected some facts, let's take a look at what you've been telling yourself about those facts.

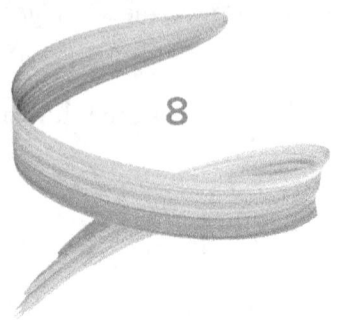

8

Who You Really Are

Who are you? I mean who are you at the very core of your being? I'm talking about your true character, the essence of your spirit.

Maybe you already know the answer. Maybe you think you know the answer. Maybe you don't have a clue.

But knowing the answer to this question is essential to finding your way through life. Knowing who you really are allows you to stop pretending you're okay and to start being who you were born to be.

So, how do you get to know yourself? Here are some suggestions to get you started.

Take a Test

I know just the word *test* can make people anxious. But taking a personality test can give you some important insight into who you are and how you relate to the world around you. Taking a test is a quick and easy way to get an overview of the "real you."

There are all sorts of personality tests, but my three favorites are the Myers-Briggs Type Indicator, the RHETI Enneagram test, and the 16 Personalities test.

You can connect with them here:

- https://www.myersbriggs.org
- https://www.enneagraminstitute.com
- https://www.16personalities.com/free-personality-test

Write about Yourself

A more personal way to learn who you are is to write about yourself. Writing in a journal regularly can help you clarify what you think and feel, and it can show you patterns in your life that you might otherwise miss.

But all that writing isn't for everyone, or maybe you're not sure where to start.

Here are five prompts to help you begin.

1. I am _____
2. I am not _____
3. People say I am _____
4. What people don't know about me is _____
5. I would like to be _____

Finding the Core of Your Character

The following exercise, inspired by one in Rhonda Britten's book *Fearless Living*, may help you see yourself in a whole new light.[7]

Please take a few minutes and read down the list of twenty-five core characteristics. Then pick the three you believe best apply to you.

(If you have a characteristic that isn't listed below, feel free to add it to your list.)

Twenty-Five Core Characteristics:

1. Accountable
2. Adventurous
3. Authentic
4. Charismatic
5. Creative
6. Collaborative
7. Confident
8. Courageous
9. Easygoing
10. Efficient
11. Fair-minded
12. Generous
13. Honest
14. Inspirational
15. Kind
16. Leadership
17. Logical
18. Optimistic
19. Organized
20. Outgoing
21. Practical
22. Perceptive
23. Principled
24. Reserved
25. Resilient

Write your top three choices here:

1. _____
2. _____
3. _____

I remember I wrote the following:
1. Honest
2. Kind
3. Creative

Name the person, living or dead, you most admire.

Write that name here: _____

Now pick the three characteristics you feel best define them:

1. _____
2. _____
3. _____

I chose Oprah Winfrey, and I listed the following as her core characteristics:

- Inspirational
- Leadership
- Principled

Now compare what you've chosen as *your* core characteristics to the characteristics you admire in your hero.

If you're like me, the lists are completely different. To be honest, I'd never dared to imagine those characteristics in someone like me. Those were qualities of someone better and braver than I could ever be. And maybe you had a similar reaction. Or maybe you've already recognized some of those qualities in yourself and this is just a reminder of who you really are.

Either way, there's good reason for you to claim some or all of those positive qualities you admire as your own.

Why?

Because we often have trouble seeing the truth of who we are since we're so focused on our negative self-beliefs. According to Lisa Firestone, PhD, clinical psychologist and director of research and education for the Glendon Association, "Our self-perception is often not based on what's actually going on in our lives, but rather on a negative internal distortion known as our 'critical inner voice.'"[8]

And I bet you know what I'm talking about. That voice tells you that you can't, you shouldn't, and you're not good enough. It's the voice that keeps you from seeing the whole truth of who you are.

So, for many of us, it's easier to see our positive qualities in our heroes because we've kept them hidden from ourselves or we've been afraid to acknowledge them. Our good qualities are mirrored back to us in the people we admire.

Take another look at that list of your hero's qualities and ask yourself if they could possibly apply to you.

What if that power, that wisdom we admire in other people, is just a reflection of our own power and wisdom?

To be honest, my first reaction to this idea was that it was ridiculous. I knew who I was, and I was none of those things. But then I thought, "What if I'm some of those things underneath all my fears and excuses?"

And when I thought more about it, I realized I might indeed have some of those characteristics, but I'd been too afraid or just unaware to see them in myself. I felt an incredible rush of both fear and freedom at the possibilities if I dared claim those characteristics as my own.

What about You?

Maybe, like me, you're thinking this is ridiculous, that you know exactly who and what you are. But what if you have some of those gifts and talents hidden under your fears and excuses? What if you haven't been able to see the truth of your strength and power? What would your life look like if you could see these characteristics in yourself as clearly as you see them in others?

Let your imagination go wild, then write about it here: _____

_____

_____

_____

_____

_____

_____

_____

Now it's your turn to write the truth of who you are.
So, write your true core characteristics:

1. I am _____

2. I am _____

3. I am _____

Now that we know who you are, let's talk about how we can go about making changes in what you tell yourself about who you are.

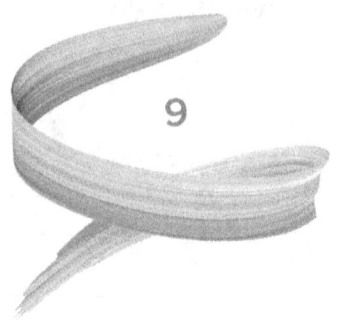

Talk about Your Story Differently

Whatever's going on with you, whatever kind of stress, fear, and anxiety you're dealing with, you can change the story you tell yourself about who you are and what you can do. This is one of the best ways I know to ease fears, and the easiest way to start is by changing the words you use to tell your story. Now, it may seem like changing a word or two couldn't make a difference. But I know from personal experience how changing just a word can change everything.

Change Your Words, Change Your Life

To get licensed as a therapist, I had to take a Big, Scary, Important National Test. I admit just the word *test* makes me nervous. I was terrified.

I spent months studying. I spent sleepless nights going over all the information I needed to know. I ate too much. I didn't eat at all. I was cranky and exhausted. And as the test date approached, I managed to talk myself into believing that I was going to fail. I convinced myself that there was too much to know. I was going to freeze up. I'm not good at taking tests. I was doomed!

I was studying hard. I knew the information, but at the same time, I knew I was talking myself into failing. And I didn't know what to do about it. I was panicked.

At that point my husband stepped in. He'd taken an Important National Test himself, and then he'd helped other people through the test-taking process. And he had the answer for me.

He said, "You need to talk about this differently. Instead of telling yourself that this is a terrible, horrible, awful experience, tell yourself that this is an adventure. Call it an adventure. Call it a challenge. Call it a once-in-a-lifetime experience. Tell yourself this is something to be curious about—not a disaster waiting to happen."

What a difference that small change made in how I felt about that test.

Being curious allowed me to shift my thoughts from my usual list of pointless, negative questions about a possible future: what was going to happen if I failed, why I'd even thought I could pass in the first place. Instead, I could embrace some rational thinking about what the test was really going to be like.

And when I imagined the truth, I was able to not only relax but to prepare for the test in a calmer, more useful way. I planned to eat well beforehand, get a good night's sleep, wear comfortable shoes and a sweater.

And when I finally sat down to take the test, I felt prepared and reasonably calm and centered.

The shift in language helped me pass the test, and that made a real difference in my life.

No question about it: When we use negative, fear-based words, we make ourselves anxious and afraid. When we change those words, we can ease that anxiety and fear.

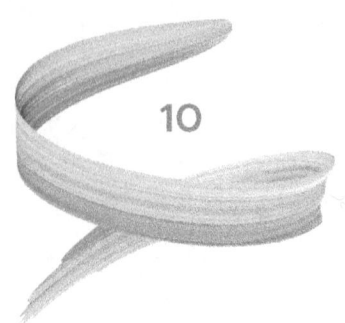

Five Simple Phrases That Can Change Your Life

Adding one or all of these phrases to your life can go a long way in helping you tell a positive story about who you are and what you're capable of doing.

1. **"I choose to" and "I choose not to."** These two simple phrases have enormous power. When you substitute them for the usual "I don't want to," "I can't," "I hate doing this," or "You've got to be kidding me, I'm never doing that," you're saying to yourself and the people around you that you've made a decision. You're making a clear choice, one way or the other.

    I struggle with going to medical appointments. And as a three-time cancer survivor, I have a lot of appointments. As nervous as I get, when I remind myself that going for the test or appointment is my choice, that changes the way I feel about going. It reminds me that I do have control in the situation. I could make a different choice, but I have the power to decide what's best for me. The phrases "I choose to" and "I choose not to" help me connect with my power. I bet they will do the same for you.

2. **"Maybe, maybe not."** This phrase comes from an old Chinese parable that has changed the way I think about all the good and bad things that happen in my life. It reminds me that things are always changing and that there's always hope. Maybe it will do the same for you. Here it is:

   Many years ago, a wise old farmer lived at the edge of a village. One day, the farmer's horse went missing. When the people of the village heard the news, they gathered at his home in the evening and said, "Oh, what a terrible loss. This is such bad luck."

   The farmer replied calmly, "Maybe, maybe not."

   The next day, the lost horse reappeared, bringing with it seven wild horses. Again, the villagers gathered at the wise farmer's house to celebrate with him. "What a wonderful gain. This is such good luck."

   Again, the farmer replied calmly, "Maybe, maybe not."

   The next day, the farmer's son was thrown off one of those wild horses and broke his leg. The neighbors gathered again in the evening to express sympathy for the farmer over his son's injury. "What a terrible accident," they said. "Your luck has run out."

   The farmer shook his head and replied calmly, "Maybe, maybe not."

   The day after that, a troop of soldiers rode into town to gather up all the able-bodied young men in the village to fight in a distant war. The son's broken leg prevented him from being taken. The people of the village gathered again to rejoice at the news. "What a blessing. This is the best luck of all," they said.

   "Maybe, maybe not," the wise old man said.

   For me, this is a powerful reminder that we don't know what's ahead. We don't know what tomorrow's going to bring, and we're often too quick to judge a situation.

What if you were able to let something happen to you without reaching a conclusion about its meaning, one way or the other?

Maybe, like me, you tend to catastrophize about what's ahead. I'm always ready to imagine the worst. But what if we could allow ourselves to be open to the possibility that something bad might happen to us—but *maybe not*. Maybe things will work. Maybe things won't be awful after all. Maybe we could think about this differently.

3. **"Sometimes."** If you're a perfectionist like me, life can be really hard. The need to do things right can make it difficult to start anything new. It can be a challenge to finish any project that isn't going well, and it can keep us locked in the fear that other people will find out we're impostors. I've found that the word *sometimes* is a real game changer for me.

    Here's what I mean: Sometimes we get things right, and sometimes we don't. Sometimes I'll succeed, and sometimes I won't. Sometimes we show up on time, finish our paperwork, or go to the dentist, and sometimes we don't. Sometimes things will go well, and sometimes they won't.

    I think using the word *sometimes* gives us permission to be human, to make mistakes, to fail without shame.

    Sometimes we're okay, and sometimes we're not okay.

    And in the end, that's what makes us human.

4. **"I will."** For me, using this phrase instead of "I can" is the difference between thinking about doing something and making a real commitment to getting it done. It's a promise to show up and then follow through. *I will* is about certainty and stepping out into the future with courage and commitment. It's the promise to yourself and the world that you can and *will* take action.

    And that matters. Because taking action is the best way I know to defeat anxiety and self-doubt. Replacing the same old what-ifs and fears with *I will* is the bridge between powerlessness and action. And even one small step forward has the power to cause a positive change.

5. **"Anyway."** One of the books that has had the most impact on my life is *Feel the Fear . . . and Do It Anyway* by Susan Jeffers. I love everything about that book, even the title. And from that title comes another word that can change your life. *Anyway* is the perfect antidote to your excuses. It asks you to stop talking yourself out of things and just get busy.[9]

Over the years I've realized *anyway* is like a magic word that helps you step out beyond your fear. It allows you to take action in spite of how you feel, in spite of what you're thinking. Remember, action defeats fear and self-doubt, and even the smallest step can make a big difference in how you think and feel. *Anyway* means no more sitting on the sidelines waiting for life to come to you. It's your ticket to the life you know you deserve.

Here's how it works:

- Be brave anyway.
- Be happy anyway.
- Allow yourself to love who you are anyway.
- Reach out to someone new anyway.
- Ask for a raise anyway.
- Ask for what you need in a relationship anyway.
- Let the truth of who you really are shine out into the world anyway.

So, let me ask you, what word or words are you using that are holding you back from living your best life?

Write them here: _____

_____

_____

_____

_____

Are there words or phrases you could use instead that would change your story?

Write them here: _____

_____

_____

_____

_____

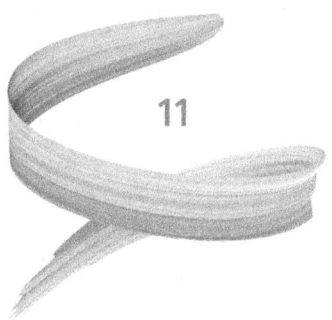

11

Letting Go of the Story of Your Past

A while back I was teaching someone to drive. We were at the top of the on-ramp of 495 and pulling into the flow of highway traffic when I noticed that my "student" driver wasn't looking at the road around us or ahead. He was looking up at the rearview mirror, staring at what was behind us. Really!

I don't remember what I said—or yelled—but I do remember being absolutely terrified and then incredibly relieved as we merged into that first lane without incident.

We were all right. But looking only in the rearview mirror, not at the road ahead, could have been a really costly error. And you know what? I think the same thing is true about the way we live our lives.

So many of us are stuck in the past. We spend our days telling ourselves the same tired stories of shame, loss, and guilt. We dwell on our failures, losses, and mistakes—in vivid Technicolor. We relive our painful moments and judge ourselves without mercy. We call ourselves names, blame ourselves for being weak and too emotional, not emotional enough, or just plain broken.

But telling those stories—and the way we tell them—is our choice. And that means we can always make another choice.

I'm not talking about changing the facts of what happened. I'm saying we can change how we look at those facts.

Years ago, I had a pair of sunglasses with pink lenses. When I wore them, the world around me looked pinker. The world hadn't changed and I hadn't changed, but seeing things through those lenses made a difference. That's what I'm talking about. Looking at the past through different lenses.

Let me give you an example.

The Story of Middle School

Middle school is tough for so many of us. Over the years, I've had all sorts of people tell me they were a miserable loser, a real loner back then. No one talked to them. The only friend they had was their dog.

What a heavy burden that story is. Imagine dragging it around for all those years. The idea that you're a loser or a loner can be devastating to your sense of self and your self-confidence. And every time you repeat that difficult story to yourself or others, you deepen that pain and the belief that you're nothing but a loner or a loser. Eventually those labels become a part of who you believe you are.

When someone would tell me a story like this, I'd interrupt by asking, "Is that really true? Is it really true *no one* spoke to you?" And invariably the story would start to change a little.

"Well, I guess the kids at the 'loser' table in the cafeteria would say hi, or that one girl in my English class talked to me sometimes, or my art teacher would ask me how I was doing."

Once they start to tell the truth of what happened, the old story might shift a little: "All right, I guess I did make some connections in middle school. I guess I wasn't completely alone, even though I've been telling myself I was."

So, at this point, the story has changed from "I was nothing but a miserable loser" to "I felt lonely and things were tough at school, but I found ways to connect. Things were tougher at home, but I found a way to feel better. I survived."

To be completely honest, middle school was not my shining hour either. But I got through it and so did you. And if we could get through *that*, I'm telling you that we're stronger, smarter, and tougher than we've been giving ourselves credit for. We're folks who went through some tough times and have learned how to take care of ourselves.

After all, we got through that tough childhood. We survived that trauma, that betrayal, that loss, that pain or shame, and we're still here. We're still standing.

So, let's start telling *that* story. Let's talk about the times we faced hardships but found a way through. The times we showed courage and heart.

Because those stories tell us the truth of who we are and what we can do with our lives.

We can begin by letting go of some of those old hurts and pains. We can work to forgive those who hurt us, and we can strive to forgive ourselves. Now, I know this is a tough conversation for so many of us. The pain can be so terrible, the scars so deep, and the idea of forgiveness so impossible. But please just hear me out. This is not about the people and circumstances that caused hurt and devastation. This is about us and healing the hurt in our heart.

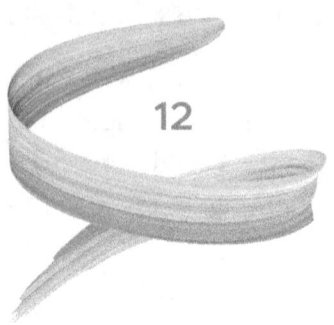

12

Forgiving

The Wand of Forgiveness

I worked as a Weight Watchers leader for years. And for all those years, I carried what I called the *wand of forgiveness* with me.

I made the wand myself by cutting out a hand-sized star from a piece of cardboard, wrapping it in tinfoil, and taping it to the end of a wooden ruler. It wasn't much to look at, but my members loved it. They were always asking me to use the wand of forgiveness because they knew instinctively that it gave them the power to forgive and start fresh without any of that guilt or shame keeping them tied to the past.

A couple of years after I'd left Weight Watchers, I was visiting a family member in the hospital when a nurse came running after me, calling my name. When she caught up to me, she said, "I need the wand of forgiveness. I've been so out of control with food. I need a new start. Can you help me?"

I told her I didn't carry it with me anymore, but I did have the pen of forgiveness with me. I took a pen out of my purse and waved it in the air and said a few words about letting go of the past—allowing her to forgive herself for any wrongdoing and start fresh. And we agreed the pen of forgiveness worked just as well as the wand of forgiveness.

What about you? Could you use the wand of forgiveness?

The Price We Pay for Not Forgiving

We pay a terrible price for not forgiving both ourselves and the people who have harmed us.

First of all, not forgiving keeps us tied to the past. It forces us to relive the trauma we suffered over and over, detail by detail, frame by frame.

Not forgiving can have a real effect on our physical health. According to Johns Hopkins, not forgiving can raise our blood pressure and impact both our heart and immune system. It can also increase symptoms of anxiety, depression, and PTSD.[10]

Not only that, focusing on the pain from our past robs us of the peace and joy possible in the present. The anger and shame we're carrying can poison both our current relationships and our relationships in the years to come.

What Is Forgiveness?

According to the American Psychological Association (APA), "Forgiveness involves willfully putting aside feelings of resentment toward someone who has committed a wrong, been unfair or hurtful, or otherwise harmed you in some way."[11]

But I see forgiveness a little differently. I see forgiving as a choice, a decision to let go of the past and move into the future without dragging that old sense of guilt, anger, or resentment behind you.

Forgiveness is something you do for yourself. Forgiveness is a gift you give yourself. Forgiveness is about bringing peace to your heart and your life.

As Annie Lamott writes in her book *Traveling Mercies: Some Thoughts on Faith*, "Not forgiving is like drinking rat poison and waiting for the rat to die." So true. Holding on to old hurts and thinking about revenge or retribution is nothing but poison for you and your body. Poison.

Forgiveness is not about trying to get an apology from the offender. It's not about excusing their behavior. It's not about trying to get the offender to change their behavior or even regret their behavior. In fact, forgiveness has nothing to do with the offender. It's all about *you* and letting go of the pain of your past.

And while we can't change what we did or what was done to us in the past, what we *can* change is the way we *think* about the past.

All right, maybe you're thinking, "You have no idea what terrible thing was done to me. I was betrayed, humiliated, violated. There's no way I'm going to forgive that offender. I'm not going to give them the satisfaction."

I want to acknowledge right here that what happened to you was awful, demeaning, unbearable, and until today—unforgivable.

Maybe what *you* did was awful, embarrassing, shameful, and until today, unforgivable.

But please hear me out. Please take a moment and just imagine what your present and future might look like if you could ease that pain.

How would it feel to no longer have to carry that pain in your heart?

How Do We Forgive?

Forgiveness begins with putting ourselves in the other person's shoes. Now I know what I'm asking here is tough. And I'm *not* saying the person who did this to you was right! What I'm asking is that you take a moment to consider their side of the story.

What if your parents were abusive because they had been abused? Maybe how they treated you was the best they could do?

What if your partner grew up in a dysfunctional family and never had a chance to see what a good relationship looks like? How could they be expected to even know how to be a good partner?

What do you know about the person who harmed you? What do you know about their life? Had they been harmed or hurt as a child? Is something difficult going on in their life? Are they dealing with an illness or stress?

Seeing the Other Side

Years ago, I experienced the worst customer service of my life. The woman who was supposed to be helping me was beyond rude. She was dismissive and arrogant. She cost me days of effort and worry. In the end, she was wrong, and not only did she not apologize, but she continued to be downright nasty to me.

I remember feeling outraged at her rudeness. I was so furious that I told everyone I could about *this woman*. She was despicable, unprofessional. If it'd been today, I might have given her a terrible Yelp review, but I'm really glad I didn't.

Because a few months later, a neighbor told me that they knew this woman well. Her only son was dying of AIDS, and she was caring for him full-time while trying to work.

Hearing *her* side of the story changed *my* side of the story. She was no longer that angry, rude woman. She was a grieving mother, struggling to show up. She was doing the best she could.

That belief allowed me to forgive and move forward without the weight of my anger.

So, let me ask you: What do you know about the person who harmed you? What's their side of the story?

Asking about them can be a powerful step toward forgiveness.

When you shift your focus from your pain to theirs, that also changes your role in the story. Because you're no longer a helpless victim. Telling the story differently puts you in a role of decision-maker and action-taker. When you take steps to forgive, or even acknowledge the other side of the story, you become the courageous hero who reclaims their sense of control and power in their own life.

But What If You're the One Who Needs Forgiveness?

What if the person you need to forgive is *you*? What if you've done something, said something, or even thought something so awful that you feel like you can't forgive yourself? The way you left a relationship? The bankruptcy you filed? The lie you told? The mistake you made? The shame you brought on yourself or your family? How the heck do you forgive that?

You forgive yourself the same way you forgive everyone else: by acknowledging that you were doing the best you could. Everyone makes mistakes—including you. (I know it's hard to admit, at least for me, but none of us are perfect.)

What was going on with you at the time? Were you afraid? Were you angry? Were you exhausted, or did you feel overlooked, forgotten?

No matter what was going on, we both know you were doing the best you could. I know for sure that we are all better, bigger, and much more than that one mistake. And it's time to forgive ourselves.

Apologize

The final step we can take on the road to forgiveness is to apologize to the person we harmed. If it's too hard or too late to do it in person, you can write a text or email. Whether you send it or not is up to you. And if you can't do it today, think about maybe doing it in the future.

If you harmed yourself, the same applies. Apologize to yourself. Tell yourself you're sorry for what happened, how you harmed yourself by overeating, drinking, drugging, not speaking up for yourself, or hurting yourself in any other way.

Just take out the wand of forgiveness, or the pen of forgiveness, wave it, and let go of that burden you've been carrying.

Forgive, and set yourself free.

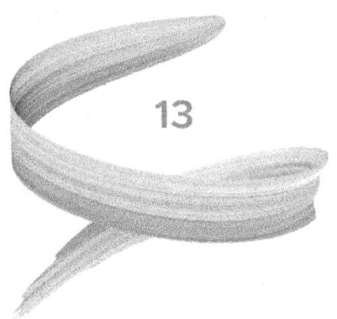

Our Story about the Future

I love playing video games. I love solving the puzzle or building the city or the empire. But most of all, I love being the hero who faces danger with courage and confidence and wisdom, knowing everything will be all right, whatever the game throws at me.

It's fun to put on the armor or pick up the wand and take on a new adventure, knowing that if I don't succeed or get what I want, that doesn't mean there's something wrong with me or that I should give up the journey. It just means I have to try another path, or find another spell, or ask another character to lend a hand. No matter what happens, I can't fail. I just press Restart and try again.

And that got me thinking. Wouldn't it be great if we could show up for the game of life like that—knowing we could meet any challenge with courage, confidence, and wisdom. What if we knew that no matter what went wrong, we could find another path or another spell, or we could just press Restart? What if we knew we would be able to handle anything life throws our way?

What would we have to be afraid of?

I don't know about you, but I can't think of a thing.

If I knew I was like that hero in the video game, I would trust myself to take care of whatever happens in the future. And that means I could stop scaring myself with all those terrible stories of what *might* happen.

Maybe you know what stories I'm talking about. Maybe you tell yourself the same kind of stories, full of doom, gloom, failures, losses, and tragedy. Stories that keep us frozen with fear and unable to sleep at night.

So, why the heck do we scare ourselves with those stories of disaster and catastrophe? I know I do it because I'm hoping that if I imagine the absolute worst long and hard enough, I'll be able to prepare for it—or head it off. And I'm guessing it's something similar for you too. I think we worry obsessively to try and control the future and to keep ourselves and the people we love safe from harm.

But here's the truth. *Worry does nothing to change the future.*

No matter how hard we worry or how anxious we make ourselves, it's not going to change anything that happens in the days ahead. That's beyond our control.

But what we *can* control is the story we tell ourselves about who we are and what we're capable of accomplishing. What if we decided to be the hero in our own story?

The Hero's Role

Instead of telling our story from the point of view of someone who's at the mercy of life and circumstance, what if we cast ourselves as someone with courage, strength, and the ability to handle whatever comes our way?

I say let's claim the role of hero!

Now, I bet you're already arguing with the idea that you could be a hero. You may even believe that role is impossible for someone like you. Well, I beg to differ. I believe you're perfect for the role of hero in your life story. In fact, I believe there is enough greatness in every one of us to make us all superheroes. I believe we all have a superpower.

What's Your Superpower?

Every hero has a superpower, and so do you.

There is something special about you, something that sets you apart, a quality you and the people around you can count on when the going gets tough.

Now, you may already know exactly what I'm talking about. You have the gift of bringing people together, or the gift of persistence, or you have a great sense of humor. If so, good for you.

Write it here: _____

_____

But if you're not sure, here are some questions to ask yourself to help you see your superpowers more clearly:

1. What comes naturally to you? Is there a talent that comes easily? This could well be your superpower.
2. What's special about you? Your different perspective, that unique view of the world? This could be your superpower.
3. What do other people say about you? What compliments, kudos, or awards have you collected over the years? If people are telling you that you have a superpower—listen to them.
4. What do people count on you to do at work? Other people may notice things you do well, things you may overlook. If they can rely on you, that's proof you can rely on yourself as well.

Write your superpower here: _____

_____

So, now that we've identified your superpower, there's just one more thing you need to do to step into that hero's role: understand the hero's secret.

The Hero's Secret

Remember a time when there was something you really wanted—a better job, a new relationship, a home of your own—but you let your fear hold you back from taking action.

Now think of someone you really admire—someone you think of as a hero. It could be a family member, a friend, someone famous, living or not. Just pick someone who inspires you!

Write the person's name here: _____

_____

_____

Imagine that person really wants something with all their heart. Something like a new job, a better relationship, a home of their own. Like you, they may be afraid. But they don't let that stop them. They do something that makes a difference.

They talk to themselves differently. Instead of scaring themselves with stories of past failures and fear, they remind themselves of strength, courage, love, trust, or adventure. They focus on what they really want and talk themselves into believing they're capable of getting it.

And it's that positive self-talk and focus on self-belief that helps them step past their fear and take action.

Because here's the truth about heroes: Heroes act. In spite of their fear.

They may be afraid or anxious, but they act anyway. They make mistakes, they mess up, they embarrass themselves, but they act anyway. Maybe they just take a small step. Maybe they do one small thing. And if they fall down, they get up again and again until they get the job done. Heroes show up for themselves and for the people around them.

It's Our Turn

And what does that mean for us? It means all we have to do to claim that hero's role in our life is to find the courage to act, in spite of how we feel, how we think, or what people tell us we can and can't do. We don't have to get rid of our fear. We just have to take a few steps past it.

Now, maybe you're thinking it's impossible to act when you feel paralyzed by fear. But like those heroes, we can learn to talk to ourselves differently. And here's a simple technique that can help us move beyond our fear.

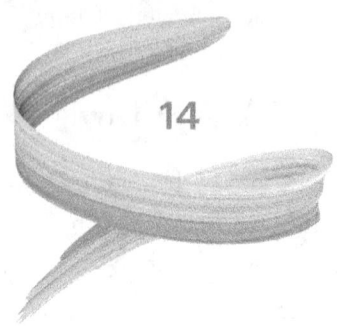

14

Act as If...

I've always loved the movie *Tootsie*. It's the story of a talented actor (played by Dustin Hoffman) who's so stubborn and hard to deal with that no one will hire him. In desperation, he dresses up as a woman to land a part in a soap opera. When he gets the part, he's forced to continue to act as if he's a woman.

Over time he embraces his new identity as a woman. He begins to listen more and relate differently to the people around him. And in the end, acting as if he's a woman changes him, making him a better actor and a better man.

By acting *as if* we already are who we want to be, we can make similar changes in ourselves.

Claiming Your Best Self

Now, I'm not talking about being fake or deceptive. I'm talking about being your true, authentic, very best self. That powerful, loving human being we both know you are. No more letting other people's opinions define you.

This is about claiming the best of you!

Acting *as if* allows us to do an end run around that loud, shrill voice of judgment in our head that tells us we're broken, we can't take care of ourselves, and we're not good enough. When we focus on what we're doing instead of what we're thinking or feeling, we can interrupt that loop of negative thinking and put down all that heavy emotional baggage we've been dragging around.

And when we put down that baggage, even briefly, it allows something magical to happen in our brains:

1. When we stop listening to that critical voice and those negative thoughts, it allows us to focus on some positive new thoughts about those heroic qualities we can rely on to create the future we've been dreaming of.
2. When we stop imagining the worst and start thinking about positive possibilities, that allows us to look for solutions to our problems.
3. From those possible solutions, we can begin to put together a road map to lead us to what we really want in life.

So, if you're ready to act *as if*, here are some simple things you can do to get started.

How to Act like a Hero

1. **Change your posture.** To act like you have the courage of a hero, you don't have to fly, change shape, or lift a building. When you're facing something that makes your palms sweat and your heart pound, all you have to do is sit or stand up straight. You may already know that when you sit up straight, you feel better physically. There's less stress on your back, your shoulders, and your neck. You can breathe more deeply and digest your food more easily. (Not to mention it makes you look five to ten pounds thinner.)

And research shows that sitting up straight can make you more confident, clearheaded, and even more optimistic.[12]

Want some proof? Go ahead, hunch over. Let your spine round and your head hang low. Slump as low as you can go and try to feel optimistic, courageous, or good about yourself.

Now, sit up straight. Square your shoulders and lift your spine. Make sure your ear lobes are over your shoulders. Notice the difference in how you feel. That's the power of posture.

So, when you're confronted with danger or fear, all you have to do to claim a hero's courage is stand up straight.

2. **Smile**. If you want to feel more cheerful, all you have to do is smile. You may think just smiling won't make a difference in how you feel. But a recent research study from the University of South Australia confirms that simply moving our facial muscles can cause our mind to be more positive. The study involved asking some students to simulate a smile by holding a pen between their teeth.

As Fernando Marmolejo-Ramos, lead author of the study, writes, "When your muscles say you're happy, you're more likely to see the world around you in a new way."[13]

So, if you want to feel better, just smile.

3. **Dress for success.** You don't need a cape to dress like a hero. All you have to do is choose to wear clothes that make you feel powerful and positive about yourself.

I think over the last few years, we've all experienced the powerful lift in energy and optimism that comes when you trade in sweats for clothes with shape, style, and a belt. So it may come as no surprise that there's science showing that what we wear has an effect on how we feel about ourselves and how confident we are in our abilities.

A study appearing in the *Journal of Experimental Social Psychology* looked at fifty-eight students, some of which were asked to wear what they were told were lab coats. Others were asked to wear the same white coats but were told they were artist smocks. The rest remained in street clothes. They were then all asked to do a number of attention-related tasks. Those wearing the lab coats did better at those tasks and made far fewer mistakes than those who were told the coats were artist smocks or those who were wearing street clothes.

Why?

As the study authors write, "Clothes can have profound and systemic psychological and behavioral consequences for the wearers."[14]

So, put on that tailored jacket, pull on those boots, or pull on the jeans that make you feel like a million dollars—and claim that role as hero.

4. **Have fun.** Remember the fun you had pretending when you were a kid? That's what I'm talking about. Think back to those early days. Maybe you played air guitar, dressed like a princess, or constructed your own planet out of LEGO blocks. Not only was all that pretending fun, but it was also great practice for adulthood. Today, acting *as if* is the same kind of idea.

Imagine what it would be like to headline on Broadway, climb Mount Everest, or move to the beach.

If you get inspired, go ahead and take a dance class, go for a hike, or start looking at real estate online.

Think of it as practice for your future. Trying out new ways to think about who you are and what you can do—just to see if they're a fit. Some will work. Some won't. If you find something that doesn't work for you, don't do it. Move on. Find the fun.

Be playful. Explore with a spirit of curiosity. No judging, no fear. Just fun.

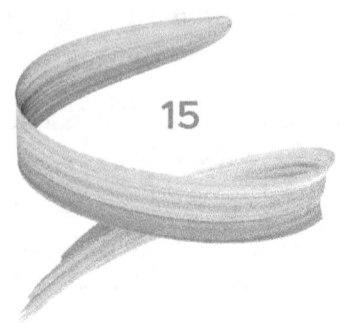

Telling the Hero's Story

When we claim the role of hero, we're no longer at the mercy of the future.

Instead our story becomes one of possibilities, opportunities, and power. This puts us in the driver's seat. From here on in, we're in charge.

No more stories about lack and loss and doom. It's time to step out beyond our fear and toward the courageous, powerful life we were born to live. Ready, set, go—and do.

Building a Hero's Future—Building Trust with Yourself

You've claimed the hero's role, and you've started telling yourself the story of what's ahead for you. But how do you keep yourself on the road to a calm, centered life?

By learning to trust yourself.

What do I mean by that? I mean you know you're going to show up, no matter what. You can count on yourself to follow through, to do your best, and to treat yourself with the same respect and care you treat others.

When you trust yourself, it means you always have a friend. You always have a safe place inside you, and you can always count on yourself to stand up during the tough times.

So, how do we build that trust with ourselves? The same way we build trust with anyone else. By being consistent, loving, compassionate, kind—and by keeping our word, no matter what.

Seven Promises to Make and Keep with Yourself

1. **Keep your commitments to yourself.** If you make an appointment with your dentist or your lawyer, I bet you show up, right? Why? Well, because you have to pay for that appointment anyway. But it's also because you value the other person's time. What if you valued your time the same way? If someone else didn't show up for an appointment with you, would you trust them? And if you consistently failed to show up for your dental appointments, would the dentist trust you? I don't think so.

    But how often do we promise ourselves that we're going to go to the gym or apply for a new job only to ignore that promise as if it doesn't matter—because it's just us, and we don't matter. Listen, no one can trust someone who doesn't keep their word. Be trustworthy. Honor your word to yourself. You deserve it!

2. **Speak to and treat yourself kindly.** No one trusts someone who's mean to them. You certainly wouldn't trust anyone who threatened you, yelled at you, or called you names. Don't allow it from yourself. From now on, only accept from yourself the same kind, supportive language you'd accept from anyone else. Period. End of sentence. (And no more judgment.)

3. **Treat your body kindly.** Take care of your physical needs. When you ignore your body's needs, you're telling yourself they don't matter. You're saying that you're willing to let your

body suffer while you take care of someone or something else. You certainly wouldn't trust anyone who abused or neglected you physically. It's time to stop allowing that from yourself. No more putting off your needs. Honor your body's needs.

When you're hungry, eat.

When you're thirsty, drink.

When you're tired, rest.

And when you need to go to the bathroom—go!

Your body is always telling you what it needs. All you have to do is listen.

4. **Speak up for yourself.** Asking for what you need is a powerful way to build trust with yourself. When you know you can depend on yourself to speak up, you don't have to be afraid that you won't get what you want. Here's the bottom line: if you don't ask for what you need, you can't expect to get it.

   Over the years I've spoken to lots of couples who've shared all sorts of stories about the odd, inappropriate, and even insensitive gifts they've given each other.

   I've heard things like, "I wanted diamond stud earrings, but he gave me a vacuum cleaner" and "I wanted a chainsaw, but she gave me exercise equipment."

   Maybe it's happened to you. It's happened to me.

   But here's the truth.

   Your partner, child, parents, coworkers, and everyone else in your life cannot read what's on your mind, no matter how much they love you.

   To get what you want, you have to ask for it!

5. **Set boundaries with yourself and others.** Practice saying no. I know, saying no can be tough for several reasons. It means you're going to disappoint people who may or may not be understanding. It means you have to make a decision about what really matters to you and what doesn't. And it means

you're going to have let go of some experiences and opportunities you might have really enjoyed.

But there's also a big payoff in saying no. If you don't do whatever it is you're saying no to, you're going to have more time and space to do the things that really matter. And in doing the things that matter, you're creating a life full of what is most important to you.

6. **Step outside your comfort zone once in a while.** There's an old saying: "Everything you want is waiting for you on the other side of your comfort zone." So true. But how do you get there? Just take one small step. And then take another small step, and then take another step after that. My mother-in-law lived with MS for over thirty years, and she made it look easy. When I asked her how she was able to live so courageously, she pointed to a sampler she had hanging beside her stove. It read: "Yard by yard, life is hard. Inch by inch, it's a cinch." She was right. It all comes down to that one small step.

7. **Let your light shine.** Talk about yourself positively. Stop putting yourself down.

Let me end by sharing my favorite saying about trusting yourself, which is by author Charlie Wardle: "A bird sitting on a tree is never afraid of the branch breaking because her trust in not on the branch but on its own wings. Always believe in yourself."

Part Three

The Fear of Change

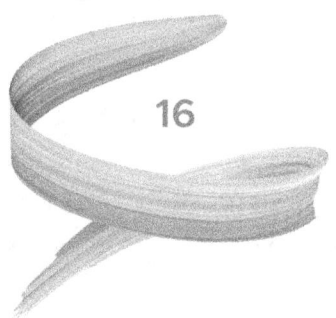

What Is the Fear of Change?

While self-doubt is often a result of the story we tell ourselves about the *past*, the fear of change is usually at the root of the story we tell ourselves about the *future*.

As Albert Einstein said, "The only thing certain in this life is that nothing is certain." And that uncertainty is a big part of what makes us anxious. We're anxious because we don't know what's going to happen.

Knowing vs. Not Knowing

I don't know about you, but when I'm reading a book, I often peek ahead and read the ending because I don't want to wait to find out how it all ends. And I love watching movies I've watched before. Why? Because if I know the ending in advance, that means there's nothing to worry about. The outcome is certain.

And it turns out I'm not alone in wanting to be certain about how it all turns out.

Since the dawn of time, humankind has tried to predict the future. Over the years, people have studied bones, birds, the sky, crystal balls, and tea leaves for answers to what's ahead. We've also turned to religion, science, and math to not only understand the world around us but to predict the future. Will it rain on Tuesday? Will that bridge hold up all right? Will the stock market crash? Will I be able to keep my job?

And we want to know for a really good reason. Because knowing what's in the future can be really important for our survival. When we know the future, we can prepare for it. We can take steps to keep ourselves safe.

If you knew there were going to be layoffs at work, you could start polishing your résumé. If you knew your car was going to break down on the highway, you could make sure you had it fixed beforehand. And if you knew it was going to rain, you could bring an umbrella with you.

If we knew what was waiting for us in the future, what would we have to be afraid of? Not much.

But it turns out that nothing about our future is certain. Nothing! There's no way any of us can peek ahead and see how it all ends. There's nothing we can do to find out how it all turns out without living through it!

So we're blindsided by those layoffs at work. We get stranded by the side of the road for hours when our car breaks down. And we get soaked when it rains.

It's the uncertainty of how things are going to change that means we can't really know what's ahead for us. And that not knowing makes us anxious!

It's no surprise that our brains thrive on knowing. Knowing makes us feel safe, like we have everything under control.

In fact, a 2016 study appearing in *Nature Communications* found that our brains would actually prefer to experience certain physical pain rather than the pain of emotional uncertainty. The physical pain is certain. You know it's coming, so you can prepare. The emotional pain is not certain, and there's nothing you can do but wait and worry.[15]

No question about it, our brains want answers. And if they can't get the answers they're looking for from the outside world, they get to work on the inside, making up stories about what *might* happen. For those of us with anxiety, those stories of danger and disaster can have a devastating effect on our lives.

The fear of change can impact our lives in the following ways:

- We constantly seek reassurance from the people around us.
- We worry constantly that something bad is going to happen.
- We have trouble making decisions.
- We double-check our work and then check it again.
- We write endless to-do lists.
- We're afraid to speak up for ourselves.
- We're afraid of trying new things.
- We're afraid to drive, fly, ride in elevators, or travel.
- We procrastinate.
- We're afraid to leave home.
- We're full of regret over the things in life that we've missed.

If some of these resonated with you, I hope you'll keep reading. Because together we're going to take a look at what causes the fear of change and what we can do to replace that worry about the future with a sense of confidence and hope.

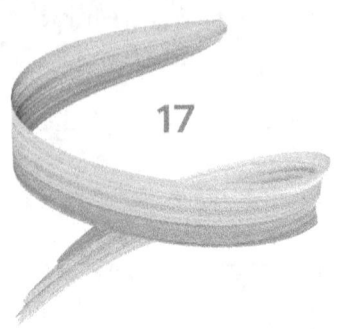

17

What Causes the Fear of Change?

Our Fear of the Dark

Think back to when you were a kid. Imagine you're lying alone in bed, staring at the ceiling. It's dark and so quiet you can hear your heart beating. And something creaks.

The breath freezes in your lungs. You can't see anything, but maybe there's something dangerous in the dark. You lie completely still, listening. What could that be?

And this is where your brain takes over and starts imagining the worst. What if there's a snake under the bed? What if there's a monster in the closet? Help!

I imagine our ancestors felt the same way as they looked out over a scary, untamed landscape, wondering what was out there. Was there a bear lying in wait? Was there a storm coming? They were worrying about how to keep themselves safe.

And I think it's the same for us today as we look into the dark uncertainty of the future. Most of us react with the same worried response because our brains are wired to fear the dark and the unknown to keep from harm. This is true whether we grew up in a safe environment or surrounded by chaos, abuse, or violence.

Part of that reaction is born in us; it's our survival instinct. But fear of change isn't just caused by genetics. Maybe, like me, you also learned to fear the future in your childhood.

What I Learned in Childhood

My family worried about everything. I mean everything. It seemed every time I left the house, my mom would warn me of some danger lurking just outside our front door. Just the way her mother had warned her years earlier.

"Be afraid." "Life out there is dangerous." "Be on your guard." "Be careful."

So early on, I got the message that life wasn't safe. And early on I learned to dread leaving the house. I dreaded going to school, I dreaded going to social events. The only place I felt completely safe was in my room, reading about life on the other side of the door and eating Saltine crackers.

I spent as much time as possible alone in my room, telling myself stories about terrible things that might happen to me or my family "out there." I made up stories of physical danger, of failure, of disaster, of embarrassment. I told myself stories of how I would never be good enough, and I certainly didn't deserve to have my dreams come true.

I made excuses and avoided as many social situations as I could. And when I couldn't avoid going, I worked hard to be as invisible as possible everywhere I went.

Over the years, I repeated those stories over and over with slight variations. "They won't like me." "I can't do that." "I'm such a failure." I repeated those stories in the belief that they were preparing me for the worst and keeping me safe. And somewhere along the way, I decided that if I worried enough about bad things, they wouldn't happen.

I believed those negative stories were keeping me safe from all the dangers waiting on the other side of that door. And over time they became a habit. Those stories were my go-to reaction to the thought of what might happen in the future.

And maybe some of this sounds familiar to you. Maybe you also got the message that life is dangerous, and you started making up disaster stories to keep yourself safe. And maybe you're still telling yourself those stories.

Or maybe it was a traumatic event or a series of traumatic events that changed the way you thought about the future.

Trauma

The word *trauma* comes from the Greek word meaning *wound*. And that's exactly what trauma is—a wound to our emotional well-being caused by some terrible and usually unexpected event.

And trauma of any kind can leave you feeling unsafe, powerless, and anxious.

Here's why:

1. Trauma causes us to lose trust in who we are and what we can to do to keep ourselves safe.
2. Trauma causes us to lose trust that the world around us is safe.

If your partner left you, you may be telling yourself the story that people cannot be trusted.

If you were in a car accident, you may tell yourself that cars are dangerous and it's not safe to ride in one.

If you've survived any kind of trauma, you may be telling yourself stories of how unsafe the world is to protect yourself from experiencing another trauma. Chances are you're making up those terrifying stories in the hope that they'll be able to keep your safe in this unsafe world.

The Negative Effect of Our Negative Stories

No matter when or why we started telling ourselves these negative stories, the truth is they are no longer serving us.

Not only that, but these negative stories rob us of peace of mind in the present. They do nothing to change the future and little to keep us safe.

What they do is make us anxious, stressed, worried, and exhausted—mentally and physically.

In fact, repeating these negative stories over and over is like living with a fire alarm that's always ringing. "Everything's dangerous!" it shrieks. "Worry about everything!"

But the good news is that we can tell those stories of the future differently. We can learn to set the alarm to respond only to emergencies, and that means we can relax and enjoy a new sense of peace in our lives.

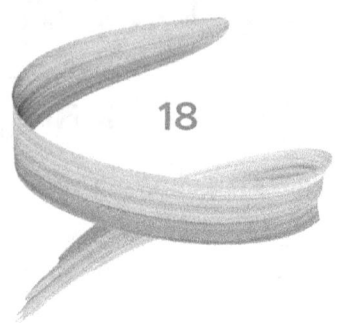

18

Giving Up the Need to Be in Charge of the Universe

Growing up, I felt it was my responsibility to make sure everyone else's needs were met, that they were taken care of—no matter what it meant for me and my needs. I was in charge. Everyone else depended on me, and that meant there was no room for error. Failure was not an option for me.

It was my job to be in control, and it still is, although I'm working on it.

Maybe, like me, you feel the need to always be in control, to be right, to be perfect, to continue your reign as Grand Poohbah of the universe. Maybe you live in fear of making a mistake. Maybe your need to be in control means you have to be perfect—or else.

But over the years, I've realized that being perfect isn't all it's cracked up to be. Sometimes making a mistake can be a good thing. Did you know that Toll House cookies, potato chips, and the Popsicle were all "mistakes"?[16] So was penicillin, the pacemaker, and the microwave oven.[17]

So, making a mistake isn't always the end of the world. And I know from personal experience that the struggle to always be perfect can come at a big price.

Take a look at the list below and see if any of these sounds familiar:

1. You judge yourself harshly and then judge everyone else just as harshly.
2. You keep redoing things in an exhausting and endless effort to "do it right."
3. You never feel satisfied with the finished product, no matter how hard you or others work.
4. You have trouble finishing things because you're afraid they won't be good enough.
5. You struggle to make decisions because you don't want to make a mistake.
6. You need to do everything yourself.
7. You value yourself only for what you can accomplish.
8. You've been accused of the need to micromanage other people.
9. You worry when your loved ones are out of sight.
10. You find other people frustrate you because they're doing it "wrong."

If you recognize yourself in any of those statements, let's see if we can figure out where this need to be perfect or right might be coming from. To do that, let me ask you to fill in the blank at the end of this sentence.

"If I'm not perfect, then _____."

Then what? What's the first thing that came into your mind? Well, that answer can be a clue to what's really going on.

Did you answer with the name of someone or some group who might be disappointed in you? Your parent or caregiver, your family, your boss? Well, maybe all your hard work is to please that person or those people. Maybe, like me, when you were young, you were responsible for everyone else's well-being. You felt the weight of the world on your shoulders, and you couldn't bear to let those people down. So, you worked extra hard to take care of everyone else, to show up for them and make their lives easier. Or maybe you lived in an abusive situation when you were young, and being perfect was a way to keep yourself or people around you from getting hurt.

Maybe you said something like, "If I'm not perfect, then everyone will know I'm a fraud" or "The world will know how anxious I am all the time, and that's supposed to be a secret" or "If I work hard enough, and I double-check my work, no one will know how anxious I am, and I can keep my shame a secret."

Wherever your need to be perfect came from, if you're tired of white knuckling your way through life and are ready to try something different, here are two suggestions:

1. **Expect less.** Go ahead. Expect less from yourself and the people around you. Lower the bar on what you need to accomplish in a day. Give up some of that to-do list. Accept that you're going to make mistakes, you're going to fail sometimes, and you're going to look just plain foolish. Acknowledge that all of that is okay. Mistakes are where we get to learn who we really are. Mistakes are where we learn how strong we really are.

    Embrace your humanness and be kind to yourself. Let's agree to stop yelling, shaming, and threatening ourselves. From here on in, let's agree that we're going to respect and support ourselves with love and compassion. We're going to treat ourselves kindly and remind ourselves that no matter how things turn out, we and the people around us are doing the best we can. And as Maya Angelou so perfectly said, "When you know better, you'll do better." Exactly.

2. **Ask for help.** The other thing you can do is ask for help. It's easy to say, but for me at least, it's really hard to do. I'm a New England girl, brought up to be fiercely independent. I

was taught from my earliest days to never, ever admit weakness or ask for help. You have to do everything yourself. And I mean everything.

When I went through treatment for breast cancer, I was, for the most part, stoic and silent about the fear that haunted my days and nights. But years later, when I went through treatment for leukemia, I'd learned better. I knew how important it was to ask for help. I went to a therapist, a nutritional counselor and an acupuncturist, and I enjoyed a weekly massage. I talked about what I was going through with friends and family.

Reaching out to others for love and support made a huge difference in how I felt and how things went. I think it can make the same kind of difference in the process of letting go of the need to be perfect.

So, if you're serious about finding ways to feel better, I suggest you join me in asking for help. Or in offering help to others who are going through a tough time. Sharing the load and walking together can make the way easier, and supporting others can give us all a greater sense of capability and purpose.

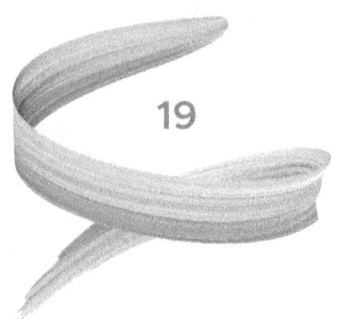

Thought Swapping

When I was diagnosed with migraines, I was told I could no longer have chocolate, aged cheese, or red wine. I didn't care too much about the cheese and the wine, but oh my goodness. Give up chocolate?

That didn't seem possible. I loved chocolate. I lived for chocolate. I dreamed about chocolate.

Hot chocolate, cold chocolate, dark chocolate, white chocolate, chocolate chips, chocolate ice cream, chocolate cookies, chocolate cereal. I loved it all.

I couldn't even imagine giving up chocolate. And then someone suggested I try replacing the chocolate with something else. Now, the truth is nothing can really replace chocolate, but when I thought about it, I realized there were some other things that might come close.

Instead of hot chocolate, a delicious latte. Instead of chocolate ice cream, coffee ice cream. Instead of chocolate chips, butterscotch chips. Instead of warm chocolate chip cookies, well . . .

All right, there's nothing as good as warm chocolate chip cookies, but I learned I really liked oatmeal raisin cookies.

And over time I found myself eating new things, exploring new flavors, and not missing chocolate at all (except for the cookies).

I realized that even though I had to give up chocolate, I didn't have to give up enjoying some delicious treats. I just had to find substitutions that tasted almost as good—or in some cases better. (I really, really like coffee ice cream). I didn't have to suffer or do without. I just had to do it differently.

I think that idea of substitution works just as well for our negative habits and thoughts.

I'm not asking you to just give up all the negative things you've been telling yourself about what disasters might lie ahead. I'm not asking you to stop scaring yourself with the stories you're making up about the mayhem that *might* happen.

What I'm asking you to do is to *replace* those negative thoughts about things you *can't* change or control with more positive thoughts about things you *can* control.

You don't have to stop your thoughts. You have to replace your thoughts.

For examples of what I'm talking about, take a look at the chart below.

Things We Can't Change	Things We Can Change
The family we were born into	The people we choose to call family
The body we were born into	How we take care of that body
Illnesses	How we choose to deal with and treat the illnesses
How other people think, feel, and act	How we feel, think, and act
The weather	How we prepare for and deal with the weather

Accidents and natural disasters	We can fasten our seat belts, install smoke alarms, and make sure we have flashlights that work.
Traffic	We can choose a different route and have extra supplies in the car in case of unexpected delays.
The past	We can control what we tell ourselves about the past and we can choose what we focus on—good or bad.
Time	How we choose to spend our time
The future	What we imagine and tell ourselves about what's ahead for us
Death	How we choose to live

So, do you recognize any of your usual thoughts in that chart? Is there one thought that you would like to replace?

Write it here: _____

What are you going to replace it with?

Write it here: _____

Or maybe you spend your time worrying about some other thing you can't change.

If so, write it here: _____

What are you going to replace it with?

Write it here: _____

All right, you've identified the thought to be replaced and the thought to replace it. The next step is to make that replacement as often as possible.

Just like ordering a latte instead of a hot chocolate, start thinking about what could go right for a change. Notice the difference in how that new thought makes you feel.

Keep at It

So, here's what I learned from my breakup with chocolate: It's tough to give up something that's been an important part of your life. I mean really tough. I would walk past a bakery, or someone would offer me a piece of chocolate fudge, and I wouldn't be able to resist. I struggled and failed—repeatedly. But I kept at it. Day after day. Over and over.

And in time, I stopped missing chocolate. I stopped thinking about it at all. Chocolate and I are over. I've moved past it. I've replaced it with some great substitutes.

It's the same with replacing those negative thoughts that you've been thinking for years. Some of those thoughts may be so ingrained that they've become a habit. When you hear rain forecasted, you always think there will be thunder and lightning and your house will be struck and burn to the ground and you will be homeless.

It's what you've always done, it's the default reaction of your brain, so replacing those thoughts will take time and patience and lots and lots of repetition. The good news is that our brains can rewire themselves with our new thoughts, so over time those positive thoughts will become the default reaction of your brain. Over time you can put an end to your relationship with those scary thoughts of doom and start enjoying a positive new relationship with thoughts of all the good things that might be ahead for you.

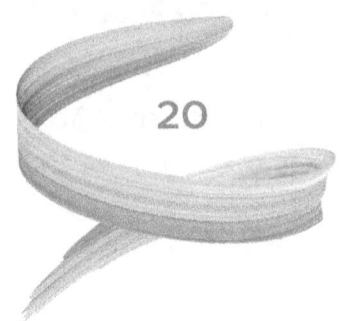

20

What Do You Really Want?

One afternoon, a man walked into an old country store. The owner was sitting on a stool behind the counter, and a dog was curled up in front of an old wood-burning stove. The owner was reading a newspaper, and the dog was whimpering and moaning.

The man stepped up to the counter. "What's wrong with your dog?" he asked the owner.

The owner looked up over the edge of his newspaper. "She's in pain," he said, and he went back to reading.

"What's causing her pain?" the man asked.

"That's been her spot for years. But recently an old nail has come up from one of the floorboards, and she's lying on it."

The man looked back at the dog and then at the owner. "Why doesn't she move?"

"Because that's where she's always slept, and that nail's not bothering her enough."

So, what about you? Are you lying on a nail? Are you complaining about your life but too afraid to do anything about it?

You're not alone! Because it's easy to complain. It's easy to point the finger, make excuses, and do nothing. It's easy to let the fear of change win. It's easy to put off what you really want for what seems easiest or least scary in the moment.

So, how do you find the courage to get past your fears and excuses?

The trick is to find a goal that's so powerful it gives you the courage to move past your fears to freedom. And how do you find that goal?

The following quiz may give you some clues about what you already love. Focusing on the things you love can help you find a path toward that inspirational goal.

And if you already have that thrilling goal, good for you. Skip the quiz and head on to the next step.

The "What Do You Love?" Quiz

1. What did you want to do when you were a kid? _____
   _____

2. Who do you envy? Why? _____
   _____

3. Where do you love to shop? Why? _____

4. What have people told you about your strengths and talents? Do you believe them? (If not, why not?) _____
   _____

5. What do you daydream about? Why? _____
   _____

6. What TV shows/movies do you love to watch? Why? _____
   _____

7. What podcasts and websites do you visit the most? Why? _____
   _____

8. What clubs, organizations, and associations do you belong to?

   _____

   _____

9. What are your hobbies? How do you spend your spare time?

   _____

   _____

10. What would you do if you had all the time and money you needed and you knew you couldn't fail?

    _____

    _____

11. Take a minute and look over your answers for clues about what you love in life. Do you notice a theme? A pattern? Something you'd like to do more of? Something you'd like to do less of? Something you need to let go of?

    Write the clues here:

    1. _____

    2. _____

    3. _____

Now, let me ask you again, what do you *really* want in this life?

If nothing big occurs to you, start with a small desire, something simple. What do you want to do this weekend? What would you like for breakfast? What kind of office chair do you really want? Start small and keep asking yourself, "What do I want now?" and "What do I want next?" The more you ask, the better you'll understand who you really are and what you really want!

Again, having a powerful goal can power you past that boundary of fear and into the life you want.

What Do You Really Want?

Write your goal here: _____

_____

_____

So now that you know what you really want, the next step is to get busy making it happen.

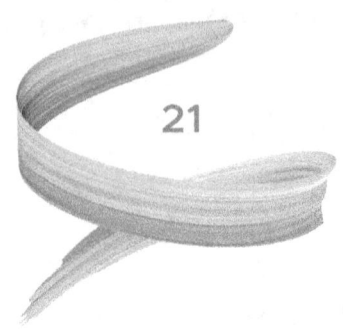

How to Get What You Really Want

A while back when my family and I were vacationing in New Hampshire, we climbed Mount Major. At least the rest of my family did—I did not. I quit halfway up the mountain, afraid to go any farther. The truth was my fear of heights kept me from finishing that climb.

Now to be completely honest, when you look up Mount Major online, you'll read that it's a family-friendly climb for folks from ages five to sixty-five.[18] No big deal, right?

Well, to me, Mount Major was a *very* big deal. It was the place I'd failed. The thing I couldn't do.

I thought about what it was like to sit alone on the side of the mountain, stopped by my fear while my family stood on the top without me.

And every time I thought about that day on Mount Major, I felt defeated.

Well, a few years later, we vacationed in New Hampshire again. And one of the things I made sure was on our to-do list was to climb

Mount Major again. I remember that even as we made the plans my hands started to sweat, and my heart pounded.

How the heck was I going to move past my fear of heights? How was I ever going to make that climb?

Now, maybe you're asking the same question about doing or getting something that you've been wanting. Maybe, like me, you've let fear hold you back from taking a single step toward that dream or that goal of yours.

So, how do we get past that fear?

Well, here are the steps I took to face my fears and that mountain:

1. **Imagine how success will look and feel.** I began by imagining what it would feel like to stand on the top of that mountain, with the climb behind me and the beauty of the view all around me. I imagined how it would feel to stand with my family, sharing that moment as a team. I imagined what the world below would look like and how amazing it would feel to know that I'd conquered my fear.

    And I didn't imagine this once or twice. I visualized it over and over, in Technicolor, with all sorts of details: what it would look like, the feel of the wind on my face, the smell of fresh air, with maybe some scent of pine. I thought about it until that picture of the goal became more real, more vivid than my fears.

    I visualized it over and over until it felt real and possible to me.

    Because the truth is that having a clear, powerful goal, one you can see and feel and taste, can inspire you and motivate you to step past your fear and anxiety to the life waiting for you on the other side.

    So, let me ask you: How would it feel to have this thing you've been dreaming about? What would it look like? How would it feel to hold the diploma in your hand? To slip your key into the front door of your new home? To board the cruise ship for your dream getaway? To see your painting in that art gallery?"

Make it vivid: see it, feel it, taste it.

And keep on imagining the thing you want until it seems real and possible and you believe you can do it! You own this.

2. **Affirm success.** The second thing I did was affirm that I could do it! Every time I thought about how difficult the climb might be, how I'd failed before, or how I hated heights, I just repeated to myself, "I can do this." There's real power in the words we use. What we say to ourselves can make a real difference in how we think and feel—and that can make a difference in what we do.

And there's science that proves it. A 2016 study appearing in *Social Cognitive and Affective Neuroscience* gives us new insight into the positive effects affirmations can have on our brains. As the authors say, "Affirmations can decrease stress, increase well being, improve academic performance and make people more open to behavior change."[19] No doubt about it, affirmations work.

So, if fear of failing, fear of messing up, or fear of anything else is keeping you from getting started along the path to what you want, find and repeat a word or a phrase that reminds you of your power, that reminds you that you've succeeded before and you can succeed again.

You can simply say, "I can do this," or "I've got this," or "I'm one powerful human being." Whatever works for you.

Here are my tips about affirmations:
- Keep them positive and in the present.
- You don't have to believe them.
- You just have to repeat them as often as possible.
- And over time, you convince your brain that they're true. You convince yourself that you *can* do it.

So, before the climb I visualized success and repeatedly said to myself, "I can do this." And that was enough to get me started climbing. But how was I actually going to get all the way up the mountain? How was I going to climb past my fears?

3. **Focus on one small step at a time.** When the climbing got tough, I focused on where I was going to put my hand next, where I was going to put my foot next. And every time I moved my hand or foot, I said out loud, "I can do this."

   I didn't let myself look up because I knew seeing how far I had to go would be discouraging. And I certainly didn't look down because I hate heights and I didn't want to demoralize myself by realizing how slowly I was going. Nope. I made that climb one small step at a time.

   "I can do this. I can do this." With every single move I made, I supported myself with that affirmation.

   And it's the same for you and your journey to the top of your mountain.

   Be in the moment. Just do one thing at a time. Don't look too far ahead, and don't look back or down. Be in the present. The present, the here and now, is the only place where we can accomplish anything. We can't get things done in the past or the future. We must be in the present for this great journey to our goal. Be focused and take it one step at a time.

4. **Don't give up. Ever.** I was about two-thirds of the way up the mountain when I stopped to rest. I pressed my back against the mountain and looked down at Lake Winnipesaukee. The view was magnificent. "Close enough," I said to myself. Because the truth was that I was terrified. I knew the hardest part was ahead, and I was trembling with a fear that kept me frozen in place.

   Then I remembered why I was there. I remembered that powerful goal. I remembered how I'd imagined it would feel on top of that mountain, surrounded by my family, enjoying the view. And I said to myself, "I can do this." I turned and reached for the next handhold on the granite and continued to climb. "I can do this. I can do this."

I did that until I reached the top of that mountain.

And let me tell you, the view from the top of Mount Major was nothing like the view from three-quarters up the mountain. Stopping short would have robbed me of one of the proudest, happiest moments of my life. Standing with my family, enjoying a 360-degree view of one of the most beautiful places on earth.

You deserve nothing less than that view.

No more cheating yourself by quitting halfway. No more giving up before you reach your goal.

If you've gotten yourself partway there, you can make it all the way there. You just have to remind yourself of what you really want—break what needs to be done into small, doable steps. And support yourself with every step you take. Don't allow what other people think of you to matter. This is your life. Don't waste it on "close enough" or "I can't."

No more quitting, no more settling.

So, my friends, this is the moment of decision. You can continue to let your fear hold you back, or you can claim that dream and make it a reality.

Just say to yourself, "I can do this," and take that first step. Because taking that first step and taking the step after that is how you get what you want.

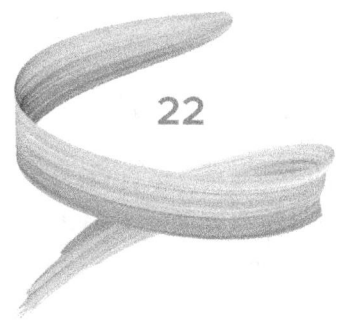

22

Travel Light
Clearing Out the Clutter

I grew up surrounded by clutter. My mom was a world-class saver of "things we might need someday." Our closets were full of clothes that no longer fit, had broken zippers, or hanging hems. The attic and basement overflowed with fondue sets, coffee makers without plugs or tops, and mismatched or chipped plates—stuff my mom was saving "just in case."

And, looking back, I realize that my mom was saving things to create a sense of safety and control in the face of an uncertain future. She could tell herself that no matter what kind of change lay ahead, if she kept those three Bundt pans, four electric frying pans, and the cookie jar with the broken lid, that would keep her and her family safe.

And I get it because I share that same feeling of safety knowing I have some extra cans of food on the shelves and extra toilet paper tucked away—ready for whatever the future might bring. Maybe you get it too.

Different Kinds of Clutter

But it wasn't just physical clutter we collected. My mom and I both clung to mental and emotional clutter as well. We hung on to our need to always be "on top of things," to achieve, to succeed, and to do it all perfectly. We held tight to old fears, hurts, failures, traumas, negative thoughts, and the certainty that something awful was about to happen. We believed that letting go of that extra waffle iron, the need to be perfect, or those scary thoughts of disaster and catastrophe would leave us vulnerable to the dangers waiting just outside our front door.

But as I've learned over the years, we were wrong. In fact, the exact opposite is true!

Clutter of any kind causes anxiety. And the more we hold on to our stuff, our thoughts, and our feelings, the more we feed our anxiety.

The Cost of Clutter

Let's take a look at how different types of clutter can affect us:

1. **Physical clutter.** At first glance, it may seem like all our physical clutter has nothing to do with our anxiety, but a small study done in 2009 found that women living in homes described as "cluttered" and "messy" had cortisol levels (a stress hormone) "associated with greater chronic stress."[20]

    In other words, being surrounded by all that mess and clutter made people stressed and anxious. (Me too.)

    While our brains are wonderful, they have a limited capacity to process information. They get distracted and overwhelmed by the piles of magazines on our ironing board and the collection of old hats in the back of our closet.[21] Then our distracted brains can't focus on what's important. Which means we have trouble concentrating, and this makes us less productive. We get overwhelmed. We procrastinate and forget things, and this leaves us anxious and depressed.[22]

2. **Mental clutter.** Mental clutter is mental overload. It's stress caused by external sources that leads to us being overscheduled, overburdened, and overwhelmed with expectations—both our own and those of everyone else.

   And that overload of information can lead to the feeling that no matter how fast we run, we're never going to get it done. No matter how hard we work, we're never going to get it right. And no matter how hard we try, we're never going to make everyone happy. And that makes us anxious.

   Unsurprisingly, a 2022 study appearing in *Current Psychology* found that the higher the overload we experience, the higher our anxiety levels.[23]

   Maybe you can relate.

3. **Emotional clutter.** Emotional clutter includes things like worry, fear, guilt, anger, grief, and even hopelessness. And I know from a lifetime of experience how tough it is to carry around that kind of emotional clutter.

   As lead writer Nikki Puccetti writes in his study published in the *Journal of Neuroscience*, "One way to think about it is the longer your brain holds on to a negative event, or stimuli, the unhappier you report being."[24]

   So, the longer we hold a negative thought or emotion, the worse we feel.

Now that we know how clutter can affect our lives, let's talk about getting rid of it.

Clearing Physical Clutter

Pick a closet, a drawer, or a room to start. Then get four bags or boxes and follow these steps:

1. Use the first bag for trash. This is the stuff you don't want and no else wants either. This one's a no-brainer. Take the bag, go

through the clutter around you, and throw out all the trash. Easy peasy.
2. Use the second bag for stuff you don't want or no longer need but that might have value for someone else. This is stuff you want to sell or donate.
3. Use the third bag for the stuff you're keeping that doesn't yet have a place. When you find something that's important enough to keep but you don't know where to put it, put it in this bag until you find a home for it.
4. Use the fourth bag for stuff you're still on the fence about. If you're not ready to get rid of it, put it in the fourth bag and wait a few months. If you haven't used it or even missed it, let it go.
5. Put away everything you decide to keep, then enjoy the sense of order and calm around you.

Clearing Mental Clutter

Do you open your eyes in the morning and think, "How am I going to get everything on that list done today?" Here are some questions you can ask to clear some of that mental clutter:

1. Do I really have to do the chore or job? Is there someone else who could do it for me?
2. What if I didn't do it right now but tackled it later in the week?
3. If I have to do it, is there an easier way to do it? Could I do part of it now and part of it later? Could I break that chore down into smaller steps?
4. What would happen if it didn't get done? Would the world end?
5. What are the three most important things that have to get done right now? Put those three things at the top of your list,

do them, and let the rest go for now. (You might be surprised at how many things end up taking care of themselves after we let them go.)

Clearing Emotional Clutter

So, how do we tackle those worried thoughts that keep us awake at night and make our days so tough? Here are the steps I suggest:

1. **Name it.** The first step to clearing emotional clutter is to give a name to what's going on with us. Is it anger? Sadness? Depression? Exhaustion? When we're able to give a name to our feelings, we create a space between who we are and what we're feeling. That space can help us step back from the feeling of overwhelm and think more calmly. Not only that, but naming your feelings can give you the language you need to learn more about them or to talk with others about them.

    But what if we're not sure what's going on with us?

    Simple. All we have to do is listen to our body—we often experience our emotional reactions physically. We talk about our "cold feet." We "shiver with fear." We have "a feeling in our gut." We feel "the weight of worry on our shoulders." So let your body tell you what you're feeling. (We'll talk more about the body later).

2. **Ground it.** Once you've named your feelings, the next step to clearing out emotional clutter is a powerful technique called grounding. Grounding works to bring you into the present by connecting your body and your mind. And today there's science to *prove* it works.

    A study appearing in *Psychological Reports* found that grounding worked better than simple relaxation to improve the mood of people with both anxiety and depression.[25]

How to Ground

The most common grounding technique is the 5-4-3-2-1 method.

It works because it makes us switch our focus away from the fearful or difficult emotions going on inside us. Instead, we must focus on what's going on *outside* us. This brings us fully into the present moment.

To use this method, begin by noticing and slowing your breath. Then do the following:

- Find five things you can see from where you're standing.
- Touch four things that are close by.
- Listen for three distinct sounds.
- See if you can smell two different scents.
- Taste one thing or remember the taste of the last thing you ate.

Visualize It

Visualization is another way to clear emotional clutter. Here's a short example:

Begin by taking a deep breath to relax.

Now, picture where in your body you feel your anger, your fear, your shame, your sadness, or whatever emotion. Put your hand over that part of your body and feel the warmth of your hand flowing into your body. Notice that the heat begins to dissolve that emotion, melting it away to nothing. You can do this as often as you'd like to let go of that emotion.

Let It Go

I know how difficult it can be to let things go when you have anxiety, but I promise you it's worth the effort. Cleaning out the emotional clutter can help you move on from some of the pain, trauma, guilt, and sadness of the past.

And finally, cleaning out the clutter creates opportunities for us to see things differently. It opens our lives to new possibilities and brings a sense of peace, calm, and order to our lives.

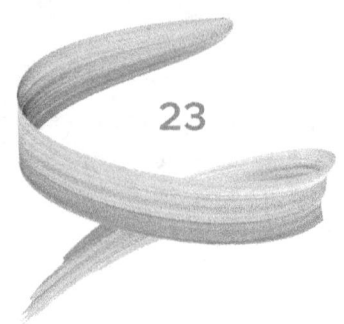

23

Birds That Flock Together
The Power of Our Relationships

The Eagle and the Chickens

Many years ago, a chicken farmer was out walking in the woods when he found a small eaglet lying by the side of the path. The farmer scooped up the baby eagle, took him home, and put him in with the chickens in his chicken coop. The eagle grew up there with the chickens and learned to walk, talk, cluck, and peck just like the chickens around him.

One day, a naturalist was driving by and was astonished to see the eagle in the yard pecking and clucking with the chickens. She stopped and went to talk to the farmer.

"You know," she said, "that eagle doesn't belong in the yard with the chickens. He was born to live in the wild, not be caged in a coop. He was born to fly, not peck along the ground. You need to let him go."

The farmer disagreed. "He's content here with the other chickens. His place is here, not in the wilderness. He would never survive."

They argued until the naturalist said, "Let's put it to the test." And the farmer eventually agreed.

The naturalist took the eagle to the top of the chicken coop and urged him to fly. But the eagle refused to leave her arm.

"You see," the farmer said.

"Let's give it one more try," the naturalist said. "Let's take the eagle to his natural environment and see what happens."

The farmer agreed. They took the eagle and drove up to the top of a small neighboring hill.

The naturalist put the eagle on her arm and held him up to the sky. For a moment, nothing happened.

"You see," the farmer said. "He belongs with the chickens."

But as he spoke, the eagle spread his massive wings and lifted up off the naturalist's arm. Then with a powerful sweep of his wings and a fierce cry, the eagle soared.

The People We Spend Time With

Our relationships shape our lives for better or worse. The people closest to us play a major role in who we think we are and what we think we're capable of doing.

And there's a really interesting study that bears this out.

The study followed the relationships of thirty-seven pairs of dormitory roommates over the course of seven months of living together. And not surprisingly, the study found that the roommates "became more similar in their emotional responses over time."[26]

So, are you hanging around with chickens or eagles? Let's take a look.

The Chickens

Take a minute and think about the people who don't support you. The people who make you feel unheard, unloved, ignored, or like a failure. You know who I'm talking about. These people ignore boundaries, won't take no for an answer, and are untrustworthy. Maybe you can think of a coworker, a family member, or even a close friend.

Write their names here:

1. _____
2. _____
3. _____

These are people you might want to try and avoid altogether, or you may at least want to limit your time with them. Their negative attitude and outlook can be infectious, and the last thing any of us with anxiety needs is to spend time with people who make us more anxious!

The Eagles

But what about the people in your life you count on? The people who make you feel better about who you are and what you can do?

Write their names here:

1. _____
2. _____
3. _____

These are people you want to spend more time with. These are the people who will cheer you on when things are going well and walk with you through the darkest of days.

Not Everyone Can Go with Us

It's important to remember that when we start making changes in our lives, everything changes, including our relationships, and that can be scary for all of us. In some cases, the people around us will welcome the changes, and our relationships with them can grow and deepen. In other cases, people may feel left out, threatened, or even betrayed by those changes. And we may find that some of our relationships no longer serve us and it's time to let them go.

If you're hesitant to let someone go, let me remind you that doing so opens room in your life to welcome new, positive relationships that support you and your healing journey.

The Secret to Relationships

Now let's talk about the people already in your life and those you're going to meet along the way. And let me tell you a secret about them, about all of us, that may surprise you.

Are you ready?

Believe it or not, those people have the same self-doubts you do. Every single one of us is afraid of something. Really. We all feel "less than" sometimes. We all doubt ourselves from time to time. And I mean all of us.

I know you're probably thinking about that famous singer, that confident politician, that self-assured actor, or that rich and brilliant CEO of a major corporation. You're thinking, "Not them! You can't tell me they're worried or anxious about anything."

But I assure you, they worry too. They have moments of insecurity. They have thoughts of failure. They've done stupid things that they hope no one ever finds out about. And they may even worry about people not liking them.

It's part of the human condition, and that's the secret. We all worry about something. We worry that people won't like or accept us. We worry that there might be something wrong with us or that someone will notice we're just pretending to be okay.

So, while you're worrying about not measuring up, know that the other person is probably worrying about exactly the same thing.

And I think knowing this can help us open up to that other person and connect with them with understanding and compassion. After all, we're in this together.

Finally, remember you are in complete control of how you show up in any relationship. No matter what the other person does or says, you get to control how *you* react. You get to choose what you do and what you say. You have the power to set boundaries, to slow things down if you feel like they're getting out of hand. And you can end the relationship if it isn't working for you. You always have the power to take care of yourself, to honor yourself in the relationship. You are always in control of *you* in any relationship.

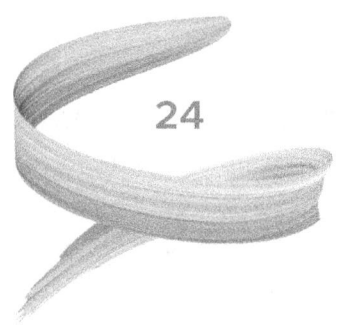

How to Handle Catastrophic Change

Finding Your Way through Fear and Panic

Something terrible has happened to you or someone you love. You're in the middle of a crisis, with no visible way out. You feel alone, exhausted, and overwhelmed. What can you do when you feel like there's nothing left you *can* do?

Let me start by sharing what I learned when I was in the hospital dealing with chemo for leukemia. I was sick, and I was scared about what was ahead. (Maybe you've been there.) I had no idea how I was going to deal with things until a social worker came into my room, sat with me, and asked me how I was doing. I told her I didn't know how I was going to get through the next few days, and she asked, "Well, how have you gotten through tough times in the past? What qualities and strengths have you relied on? What did you do? What tools did you use? If they worked before, do you think they'd work now?"

I remember being really surprised at her questions.

This was a complete switch from what I'd been thinking about. I'd been focused on how weak and powerless I felt. But when I thought back to times in my life when I was able to reach out and connect with other people, I remembered how I'd been able to rely on them and their kindness. I remembered I was good at finding humor in situations, and I always had the power to choose what I was focusing on.

Aha! I felt as if someone switched on the light. I suddenly realized that I had what I needed to get through. That switch, that change in focus and thinking, made such a difference for me.

So, let me ask you: How have you gotten through the tough times before? What qualities have you relied on? What strategies or tools did you use? Do you think any of those things would work now? If so, why not give them a try? No matter how tough things get, there's always something you can do, even if it's simply changing the things you say to yourself. You have everything you need to get through this. You just have to remember and focus on that!

When you're suffering, one of the most powerful things you can do is decide you're going to treat everyone with profound kindness—starting with yourself. Because you matter, and so do the people around you. You all deserve to be treated with respect, kindness, and understanding. Here are some quick ways to start:

- Say please and thank you.
- Share your feelings openly—listen to others in return.
- Ask what you can do to help others.
- Be honest about what you need from others.
- Ask yourself what you need in the moment to feel better. Listen and honor that need.

Remind yourself that you're doing the best you can in this situation and so are the people around you.

This Is the Most Important Thing I've Ever Learned about Getting through a Tough Time

I was just starting six months of chemo for breast cancer and was again wondering how I was going to make it through when I heard Captain Scott O'Grady's story.

He was an air force pilot shot down over Bosnia in 1995. He parachuted behind enemy lines. When the enemy found his parachute, they came hunting for him. Scott covered himself with dirt and lay still as the enemy walked within a few feet of him, shooting their rifles randomly. He was on the ground there for six more days before he was finally and dramatically rescued.

When asked how he got through such a terrible experience, he said it was what he'd learned in survival school. They'd taught him to eat bugs and leaves, but more importantly, they taught him to take things one hour at a time. That resonated with me.

"Just do your best for one hour. Don't worry about next Thursday, or 2080. Just do your best in this hour, and the rest will take care of itself."

That's what got me through chemo and the surgeries. That's what still gets me through tough times. One hour at a time.

Finally, know that this will pass. No matter how difficult this time is, it will end. Things will get better. As the old adage says, "Not to worry, not to fret. All is well, but not just yet."

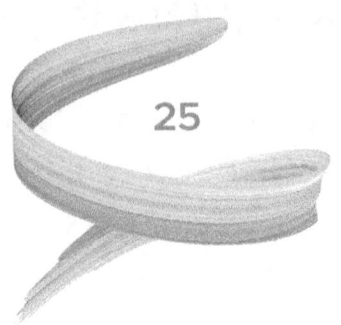

The BEAR Technique to Stop or Prevent Panic Attacks

> **Important:** If you're experiencing any physical symptoms of a panic attack, please check in with your health care provider immediately. It's important to rule out any more serious physical conditions before proceeding.

While it can be helpful to *think* about things differently, sometimes that's just not enough. And that's why I created the BEAR technique to help people deal with that panic holistically—physically, mentally, and emotionally.

Let's face it: panic attacks are tough. They can be devastating, debilitating, and terrifying. In fact, just thinking about a panic attack can cause you to have a panic attack.

No wonder people can feel helpless and hopeless in the face of their fears. No wonder they feel like there's nothing they can do to feel better.

But I want you to know you are not at the mercy of panic, no matter how real and overwhelming it may seem. There's something powerful you can do to ward off a panic attack or to stop one in its tracks.

The four simple steps of the BEAR technique are easy to remember and simple to do. There's no right or wrong way to do them. So, please experiment to find the way that works best for you.

The Four Steps of the BEAR Technique

1. **Breathe in.** As soon as you notice a sense of panic, immediately shift your focus to your breath. Notice the cool air as you breathe in and the warmer air as you breathe out. Then, as you continue to focus on your inhale, let your breath go deeper into your belly, feeling your stomach expand with each inhale as if you're blowing up a balloon.

2. **Exhale.** Now move your focus to your exhale. Because while the inhale of that belly breath is important, it's your exhale that works the magic. That exhale activates the vagus nerve and the peace-bringing parasympathetic system while silencing the red alert of your sympathetic system. (We'll talk more about the vagus nerve later.)

    *It's important to note that the more anxious or panicked you're feeling, the faster and harder you're going to want to exhale. If you're dealing with full-blown panic, you're going to want to exhale through your mouth with a whoosh. That whoosh it the real panic-buster.

    Please note: Doing this exhale more than twice can cause dizziness. If you feel at all dizzy, stop. Wait until you're feeling better before you continue.

    Continue to exhale through your mouth, but this time make the sound "ahhh." If you're feeling a lower level of anxiety, you can start with this easier exhale and continue until you feel your body relax.

3. **Affirm.** As your breathing helps ease the fear response in your body, affirm you are safe and secure in the moment.

Remind yourself that all is well and notice that the panic is already passing.

Close your eyes and imagine that your panic works just like waves washing up on the beach. Those first waves rush all the way up the beach, covering the sand. But imagine that the tide is going out and the next wave will come in with less force. It will cover less distance. And every wave after that will come in more slowly and cover less and less of the beach until the tide goes out and your anxiety eases.

4. **<u>Relax</u>.** As you continue to breathe and watch the waves of your panic recede, let your body relax. Let go of the tension in your jaw and your shoulders. Allow your body to just let go and then feel a sense of peace and ease flow through your body, your mind, and your spirit. Ahhh.

So, that's the BEAR technique. You can use it anytime and anywhere if you have a panicky thought or feel that sense of panic come over you.

But if you're feeling extreme panic, or you want to add to the power of the BEAR technique, there's one more thing you can do, and that's to add the BEAR hug.

The BEAR Hug

The BEAR hug can be used as part of the BEAR technique. But used on its own, it's also a great way to ease tension and worries and help you relax fully into a good night's sleep. I think of it as a self-hug.

Using the BEAR Hug

Begin by just getting comfortable. Take a deep breath and relax. Now cross your arms over your chest and lay your hands flat against your upper chest. Chances are your fingertips are resting on the acupressure point on your chest called the *letting go point*. It's located in that divot about three finger widths below your collarbone. Once you've found it, gently press or massage those powerful acupressure points with your two fingers.

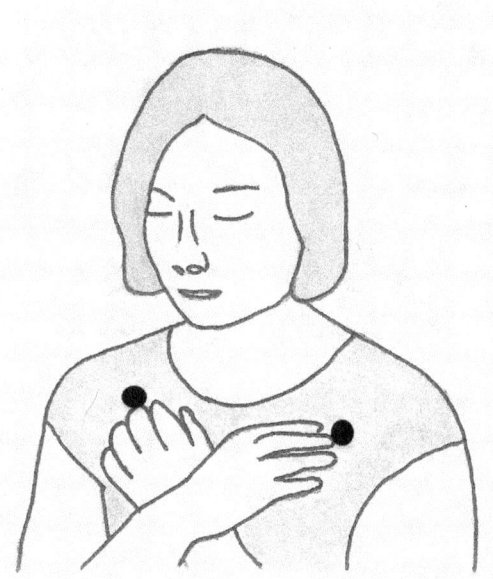

I've found that massaging these points is a wonderful way to let go of anxious, panicky thoughts. The self-hug offers an extra feeling of warmth and safety.

Part Four

Physical Anxiety

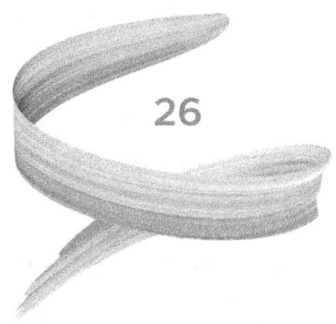

26

What Is Physical Anxiety?

It's Not All in Our Heads

So far we've talked about how our brain makes our body anxious. But if you've ever been late to an important appointment and then gotten stuck in traffic, or if you've heard footsteps echoing behind you as you were walking down a dark, lonely alley, you know that anxiety isn't just "all in our head." It's in our body as well.

Let's Get Physical

Although we tend to think of anxiety as something mental because of all those negative thoughts, our body also plays an important role in our anxiety. What we think can have a real impact on our body, and what we do and feel with our body can have a real impact on our brain. While our negative thoughts can cause all sorts of symptoms in our body, negative sensations in our body can go straight to our brain. The brain "hears" the body and responds with a whole list of negative thoughts.

Maybe you've said, "Gee, I'm not sure. I just have a feeling something's wrong." That sense is your body talking to your mind, saying,

"Something could be wrong here. You better get ready to do something about it." And the brain responds by imagining the worst.

It's a Two-Way Street

It turns out there's an ongoing conversation between your body and your mind. There's a two-way flow of information about what's going on inside you, how you think and feel about it, and what you're going to do.

Brain to body.

Body to brain.

But just how does this conversation happen? How do the body and brain talk to each other? It's starts with the autonomic system.

The Autonomic System

When I think of the term *autonomic system*, I always think of the word *automatic* because that's the perfect definition of what the autonomic system does. It's in charge of all those *automatic* body systems that keep us alive: our heartbeat, our breathing, and our digestion. It's also in charge of finding and reacting to any and all threats of danger.

You don't have to think about making your heart beat faster when you find a snake in your closet. (Or in my case, when you just read the word *snake*.) You don't have to make yourself feel like you're going to throw up before you rise to speak in public. It just happens. And that fear response not only spurs us to take action, but it also gives us an important clue as to how physical anxiety happens and what we can do to ease it.

Our Stress Response—the Gas Pedal and the Brake

Let's begin by looking at what we once believed were the two parts of the autonomic system: the sympathetic nervous system and the parasympathetic nervous system. These two systems work together to bring balance and harmony to the body.

The Sympathetic Nervous System (SNS)—a.k.a. the Gas Pedal

I think of the sympathetic nervous system (SNS) as a kind of gas pedal for the body. This part of our nervous system is all about action. It's responsible for activating the fight-or-flight response in reaction to any emergency, real or imagined.

When activated, the SNS makes our hands sweat, our jaw clench, and our legs tremble. Its job is to keep us safe. And it takes that job very seriously.

Helpful hint: I used to have trouble keeping the sympathetic and parasympathetic nervous systems straight, so I nicknamed the sympathetic nervous system the *stressful nervous system*—and for good reason. It's what causes that stress reaction.

The Parasympathetic Nervous System (PNS)—a.k.a. the Brakes

I think of the parasympathetic nervous system (PNS) as the brakes of our body. Its job is to bring a sense of peace and relaxation. When you sink into your comfy chair with a deep sigh of relief and your body relaxes, that's your PNS at work. When you're singing in the shower, dancing with your partner, or deep in soothing meditation, your PNS is in charge.

Helpful hint: I nicknamed this part of the nervous system the *peaceful nervous system* because it serves as a kind of peacekeeper for your body.

As I said, it's the job of these two systems to work together to keep our body and our mind in balance. But here's the kicker. Only one part of our autonomic nervous system can be in charge at a time. As Ellen Vora, MD, writes in her book *The Anatomy of Anxiety: Understanding and Overcoming the Body's Fear Response*, "The stress and relaxation processes are mutually exclusive. Our nervous system can't do both at the same time."²⁷ So, either the SNS is in charge or the PNS is ruling the roost. One at a time!

Now our SNS isn't always the bad guy. It was our SNS that kept our ancestors from drowning, freezing, or being eaten. And even today it serves an important function. It's keeping us alert to threats of physical danger, making us jump out of the way of an oncoming car, or prompting us to run from flames or floods.

But today, not all danger is physical. We're not usually running from bears or tigers. We're dealing with the IRS, divorce, and root canal surgery. And because our worries tend to be chronic and seemingly without end, it can feel like the sympathetic nervous system is in charge most of the time. As long as it's engaged, our brain can feel stuck in that feedback loop of negative thoughts happening in reaction to our physical stress.

And because the SNS automatically reacts to our negative thinking or to the mere thought of trouble ahead, it can make our body tense. And so round and round we go in a vicious circle.

Help!

It can seem like we're at the mercy of that gas pedal. It feels as if it gets pressed at the first hint of danger or worry and stays on as long as we're worried or afraid. And it can feel like there's nothing we can do about it.

If only there were a switch we could use to turn off that stressful nervous system and let the peaceful nervous system take over.

Well, guess what? There is!

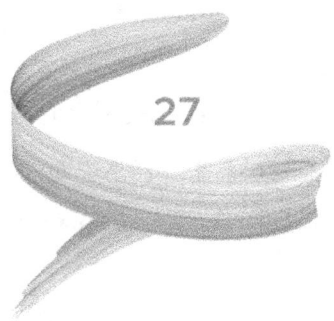

27

It's the Vagus, Baby

I think of the vagus nerve as a kind of super-communication highway that connects our body and our mind. This superhighway carries messages from the brain to the body and back again, allowing them both to work together and to respond to what's going on inside us and outside us.

The word *vagus* comes from Latin and means *wanderer*, which is the perfect name for it. The vagus nerve originates in our brain and then wanders down through our neck into our body, connecting our brain with our major organs.

But here's what surprised me: I thought the vagus nerve would be a way for the brain to give the body instructions, but it turns out it's the other way around. According to psychiatrist Ellen Vora, MD, "About 80 percent of vagus nerve fibers are afferent, meaning they gather information from the inner organs—such as the gut, liver, heart and lungs—and deliver the news about the state of affairs to the brain."[28]

And that means the vagus nerve serves to connect our two brains. Yes, I said two brains.

Introducing . . .

The Second Brain

Research shows that we have a kind of brain in our gut that's often referred to as our second brain because it plays such an important role in how we experience life.

According to Johns Hopkins, this "brain in our gut" comprises "two thin layers of more than 100 million nerve cells lining your gastrointestinal tract."[29]

And while this second brain isn't going to help you write the great American novel or remember where you put your glasses, it plays an important role in how you *feel* about things.

The vagus nerve serves as a kind of informational hotline between those brains, allowing for the flow of information and hormones between them. In fact, 95 percent of our serotonin (a.k.a. the feel-good hormone) is made in your gut, and then that serotonin travels from the gut to the brain via the vagus nerve.[30]

But that's not all. And this is where it gets exciting.

We used to believe that there were two parts to our autonomic system: the SNS and the PNS. And since only one could be in charge at a time, we would be either in a state of stress or peace.

The Revolution

But in 1994, Stephen Porges, PhD, psychologist and neuroscientist, first proposed the polyvagal theory. He suggested that the vagal nerve has two separate branches. In other words, there are two parts of our ANS: the dorsal vagal complex and the ventral vagal complex. Each has separate functions and each originates in a different location. And his polyvagal theory changed not only the way we think about the vagus nerve, but the way we think about how anxiety and PTSD show up in the body. This changed everything.

The Power of Three

So, according to Porges, there are really three parts of our autonomic nervous system:

1. There's the sympathetic nervous system (SNS), which is that fight-or-flight reaction to stress.
2. There's the ventral vagal complex, which is what we traditionally thought of as the PNS response of relaxation, calm, or the "rest and digest" response.
3. There's the dorsal vagal complex, which is the new addition, and it adds a deep new understanding about our response to stress. The dorsal vagal complex offers us a second adaptive behavior strategy beyond the fight-or-flight response of our SNS.[31]

Porges suggests that the dorsal vagal complex actually works to slow us down, or freeze us in place. I always think of the phrase "like a deer in the headlights" when I think of this reaction. This reaction can leave us feeling numb, depressed, or even hopeless. This type of reaction is often associated with PTSD, where we shut down completely to survive the traumatic situation.

The best explanation of this theory I've ever heard comes from Stanley Rosenberg's book, *Accessing the Healing Power of the Vagus Nerve*.

The Goldilocks Principle

Rosenberg uses the story of Goldilocks and the three bears to explain Porges's theory. Goldilocks was wandering in the woods feeling hungry and tired. When she came to a cottage, she let herself in. There were three bowls of porridge sitting on the table, and when Goldilocks helped herself, she found one too hot, one too cold, and one just right. It was the same with the beds. One was too soft, one too hard, and one just right.

And it's the same way with our autonomic systems:

- Our stressful nervous system (SNS) is too hot and hard. It's always looking to fight or flee from danger.
- Our dorsal vagus complex is too soft and cold. It's always shutting down or freezing in the face of danger.
- But our ventral vagus complex gets it just right by activating our peaceful nervous system (PNS), which allows us to relax, "rest and digest," or "tend and befriend."[32]

So if we're looking for a sense of calm, all we have to do is activate that vagus nerve complex. So how do we do that?

Activating the Vagus Nerve

We're going to talk more about activating the vagus nerve in the pages ahead. But here are two really powerful exercises taken from Stanley Rosenberg's book to get us started. I know they sound deceptively simple, but doing them over time can really help bring a sense of calm into your life.

The Basic Exercise

Here are the steps that Rosenberg recommends:

1. Lie on your back. (You can try this the first few times you perform this exercise, but I've found you can do it sitting or standing just as easily. It's up to you.)
2. Interweave your fingers, then clasp your hands behind your head.
3. Now, without moving your head, look to the right.
4. Continue looking right until you swallow, yawn, or sigh—all signs that your autonomic system has relaxed.
5. At this point, return to your starting position.
6. Repeat on the other side.

The Trapezius Twist

This exercise is simple and fun to do. But don't let its simplicity fool you. This is a real tension-buster, and it can be done either standing up or sitting down. Here are the steps:

1. Stand or sit up straight. Take a deep breath and grab hold of both your elbows.
2. With your elbows at your waist, gently twist from side to side for about five seconds. As you move, notice how the tension drains out of your muscles. Feel the relaxation in your body. Notice how your body is letting your brain know that everything's all right. Feel your brain relax.
3. Now raise your elbows to chest level and continue twisting for another five seconds.
4. Raise your elbows above your shoulders and twist for five more seconds.[33]

That's all there is to it. Fun and easy. Do it alone, do it with others. This is great to break up a long day at work.

So, now that we've talked about how physical anxiety works in our body, we're going to take a look at what causes it and how to ease it.

Please feel free to try as many of these techniques as you wish. See what resonates with you. If one doesn't work, go ahead and try something else. As always, this is about finding what works best for *you*! There's no right way, no wrong way, just *your* way.

So, turn to the next chapter and take a closer look at how body-induced anxiety may be impacting your life and how we can bring some new energy into your vagus nerve.

Trapezius Twist

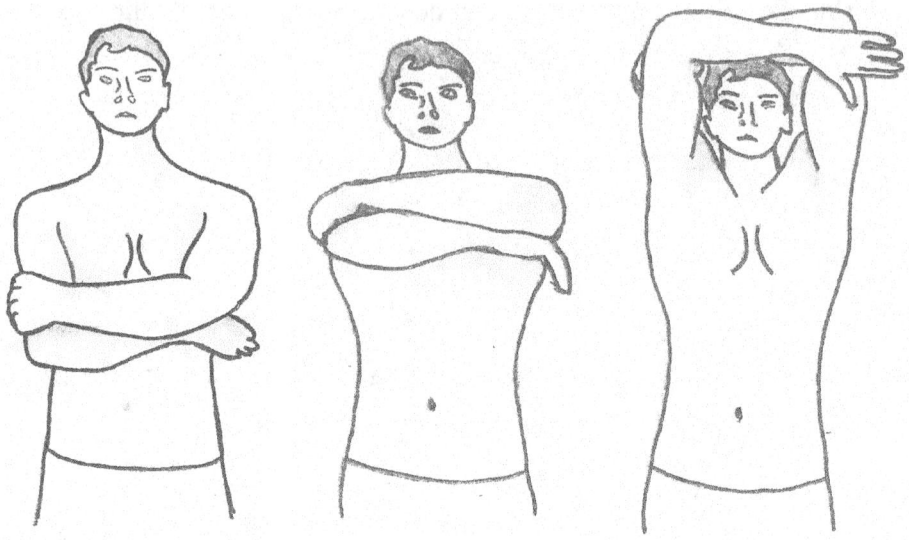

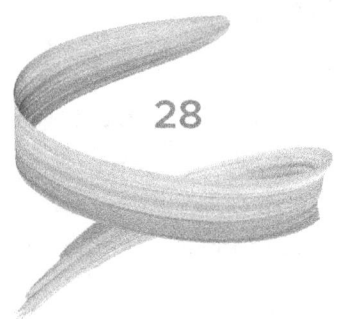

What Causes Physical Anxiety?

Physical anxiety can play a major role in our fears, and it has a number of causes. Some are evident, but some may surprise you. As you read through the list, see if any of these resonate with you.

Medical Conditions

Anxiety can be the result of an underlying health issue. A great place to start your journey to feeling better is to check in with your health care provider to see if your anxiety might be caused by some medical issue. Here's a list from the Mayo Clinic of medical concerns that might be making your anxious:

- Heart disease
- Diabetes
- Thyroid problems, such as hyperthyroidism
- Respiratory disorders, such as chronic obstructive pulmonary disease (COPD) and asthma
- Drug misuse or withdrawal

- Withdrawal from alcohol, antianxiety medications (benzodiazepines) or other medications
- Chronic pain or irritable bowel syndrome
- Rare tumors that produce certain fight-or-flight hormones[34]

Drugs

According to WebMD, a number of medications can make us anxious. Drugs like corticosteroids, asthma medications, thyroid medications (I know about this one personally), ADHD medications, seizure medications, and medications containing caffeine to treat headaches and migraines can make us anxious.[35] If you're taking any of these, you might want to check in with your health care provider to make sure you're on the right track.

Genetics

I come from an anxious family, and maybe you do too. So, is our anxiety genetic or learned? Probably a little bit of both.

We've already talked about the major role both our childhood and trauma play in making us anxious. But there's no question that genetics play a role as well. The question is how much of our anxiety is nurture and how much is nature.

The truth is that we don't know. Lots more research is needed before we have a clear understanding of how genetics and environment work alone or together to make us anxious.

But here's what the science tells us today:

- A 2017 study found that if one of your parents has generalized anxiety disorder (GAD), you have about a 30 percent chance of having it too. So if, like me, your mom was always anxious, you may be as well.[36]

- Research also shows that if a close relative has panic disorder, you're three to five times more likely to have panic disorder yourself. Again, if your sister has had a panic attack, you may have one as well. But maybe not. While genetics may play a role in our anxiety, it's only one factor in who we are, what we are, and what's ahead for us.[37]

Lifestyle

You're probably aware that how we care for our physical body has a real effect on our anxiety. Most of us know that eating a healthy diet, performing some daily exercise, avoiding caffeine, and getting a good night's sleep can help ease anxiety. But there are some other important aspects of our daily life that can impact how we think and feel.

As we've discussed, our social connections are critical to our mental health, and so is our environment. Clutter can make us feel anxious and overwhelmed. But that's not all. A 2021 study in *Lifestyle Medicine* found a number of other factors that can play a role in how we feel. See if any of these resonate with you:

- Worrying about money and financial security can create a real sense of fear in our lives.
- Spending only a few minutes a day getting some fresh air can help ease our anxiety.
- Having an animal in your life is a powerful way to reduce stress, although it's not for everyone.
- How much time we spend looking at screens can play a major role in how we feel about ourselves and our life.[38]

Our Thoughts vs. Our Emotions

I see our thoughts as a kind of nonstop internal monologue in reaction to the world around us. "I like this time of year." "I should call my grandmother." "Where are my glasses?" "What's wrong with me?" "Why can't I be like everyone else?"

And these thoughts lead us to make decisions about how we should act and how we should feel. There's a lot of power in our thinking, but it's our *emotions* that show up in our body as sensations and symptoms. We don't just *think* our emotions; we *feel* them in our guts, our shoulders, our racing or broken heart, our shivery spine, or our sweaty palms. So those physical symptoms we experience are a result of how we *feel*.

It's our emotions that cause our physical anxiety, not our thoughts. When we feel nervous, unhappy, or fearful, our body answers with all those physical symptoms.[39]

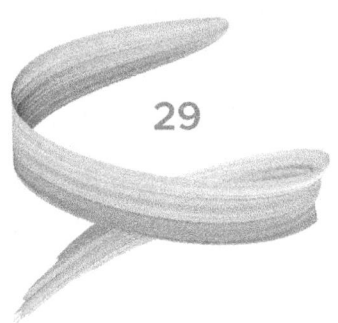

The Price We Pay for Physical Anxiety

> **Important:** These symptoms of anxiety can also be symptoms of a number of medical conditions, so it's important that you check in with your health care provider first to rule out any physical conditions.

Physical anxiety shows up differently for all of us. But if you're experiencing any of the following symptoms, you may have body-induced anxiety.

Physical anxiety can cause the following:

- Trouble sleeping
- Digestive problems of all kinds
- Chills and/or sweats
- Numbness or tingling in your hands and feet
- Headaches and/or dizziness
- Heart palpitations and chest pain that can mimic a heart attack
- Uncontrollable trembling or shaking
- Exhaustion

- A tightness in your chest that makes it hard to breathe
- Unexplained muscle pain

But such symptoms are just part of the impact physical anxiety can have on our lives.

Health

While our bodies are equipped to handle the physical effects of stress in the short term, long-term, chronic stress can have a serious impact on our bodies. According to the APA, "Stress affects all systems of the body including the musculoskeletal, respiratory, cardiovascular, endocrine, gastrointestinal, nervous and reproductive systems." And over time stress and worry can lead to high blood pressure, heart attacks, strokes, high blood sugar, a host of GI concerns, and issues with your immune system that can leave you at risk for other health conditions.[40]

Work

Physical symptoms may keep you from showing up at work. And if that's the case, you're not alone. According to a 2022 Gallup survey, "19 percent of US workers rate their mental health as fair or poor, and these workers are four times more likely to call in sick. And that adds up to almost 12 sick days. Over the course of a year, all those absences cost the economy $47.6 billion dollars in lost productivity."[41]

Fear of Fear

Here's a term you may have never heard before, but it can wreak havoc in our lives: *anxiety sensitivity*.

What is it?

According to an article from Harvard Health Publishing, "Anxiety sensitivity is a tendency to misinterpret the sensations that accompany anxiety—irregular breathing, heart palpitations, trembling, flushing, sweating, stomach rumbling—as indications of imminent physical danger or serious illness."[42]

We worry that our racing heart means we're going to have a heart attack, or we think feeling dizzy might mean we're going to have a panic attack. And we're terrified these symptoms might cause us to lose control, and then other people will see and judge us. Just the thought of the possible embarrassment or loss of control can be enough to keep you a prisoner in your home, feeling trapped and lonely, longing to be able to join in life.

In other words, just the thought of experiencing those physical symptoms in a public place can make us afraid to leave our homes and keep us from showing up in our lives. They can cause us to miss important events and special moments—weddings, graduations, funerals. They can keep us from maintaining relationships with our friends or meeting new people. And they can make us downright miserable.

But the good news is there are some really positive ways to deal with our physical anxiety. And in the next chapters, we're going to take a look at things that can make a real difference in helping us feel better.

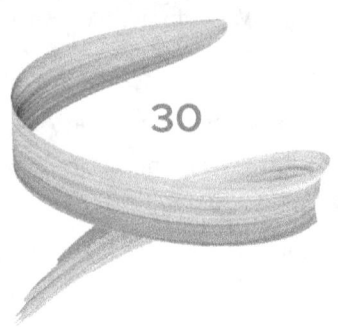

Just Breathe

I don't know about you, but there are times in my life I get so trapped in a downward spiral of worried thoughts that it's clear I can't *think* my way out.

At that point, I know the one thing I can do is *breathe* my way out.

Why It Works

Since the dawn of time, humankind has used their breath to still their minds, calm their bodies, and bring peace to their souls. And today we have a much clearer understanding of how and why this works.

As I mentioned earlier, our breathing is controlled by our autonomic system, and that means we breathe automatically, similar to the way our heart beats, our blood circulates, and our food digests. It all happens without any input on our part.[43]

But unlike those other functions, *we can control how we breathe.* And because we can control how we breathe, we can change the way we breathe anytime we choose.

According to a 2017 study, when we slow our breathing, it "causes a shift to our parasympathetic dominance and increases our vagal tone." And that puts our parasympathetic system (peaceful) in charge, which allows us to ease into a state of relaxation.[44]

It sounds simple enough, but if you're like me and you get overwhelmed with feelings of fear or panic, changing your breath may feel impossible at times. So, I've broken the process down into three simple steps you can take anytime you want to create a sense of calm in your life.

1. **Go slower.** Begin by just noticing your breath. Chances are if you're stressed or overwhelmed by fear, your breathing is fast and shallow. To change that, take one long inhale through your nose, then exhale through your mouth with a whoosh. Continue to focus on breathing ever more slowly. That's all. Just make one breath after the other slower and slower.

   And as you slow your breathing, notice how your heart rate slows, allowing your body to relax and your fears to ease.[45]

2. **Go deeper.** The next step is to allow your breath to flow deep into your belly. Then as you continue to breathe deep into your belly, focus on expanding your ribs. I think of it as *balloon breathing* because it's like we're blowing up a balloon in our belly and then letting the air out.

   But whatever you call it, this kind of deep breathing not only brings a sense of relaxation to your body, but it also lets your brain know there's nothing to worry about and it's time to take it easy. Both your brain and your body can relax a little. I bet you'll find that doing this regularly will make a real difference in how you cope with your fear and worry.

   Today's research backs this up. According to a 2010 study, deep abdominal breathing works to reduce the sympathetic (freeze, fight, or flee) response and at the same time enhance vagal activity.[46]

3. **Go longer.** This third step is something I've found to be a real game changer. Focus on and lengthen your exhale. Let's try this together to see how this works.

- **Breathe In**

    Go ahead and inhale. As you breathe in, do you notice that your body tenses a little? Maybe you feel your shoulders lift and your heart beat a little faster.

    From our first breath on this planet, our inhale has activated our sympathetic nervous system (stressful nervous system), and this has called our bodies into action. You may have noticed that when you're stressed, in danger, or just surprised, you breath in as your body gets ready to fight, flee, or freeze.

- **Breathe Out Longer**

    All right, now exhale. As you breathe out, do you feel your shoulders softening? Can you feel your body relaxing? That's because when you breathe out, you're activating your parasympathetic nervous system (peaceful nervous system), allowing your body to rest.

    And when we sigh or yawn, we are again activating our vagus nerve, putting our PNS in charge.

- **Focus on That Exhale**

    When you focus on the exhale, you activate the calming part of your nervous system and so ease your anxiety. The longer and slower the exhale, the calmer you'll feel. It sounds simple, but boy is it powerful.

    So, there you have the three steps for using your breath to take you from panic to power. But maybe you're looking for a more formal breathing practice, something you can do daily to feel better in the moment and to build a foundation of long-term calm in your life.[47] You can find a few options below.

The Coherent Breath

The coherent breath is my absolute favorite go-to breath for creating that deeper sense of calm in my life. It comes from the book *The Healing Power of the Breath* by Richard P. Brown, MD, and Patricia Gerbarg, MD, and they recommend this breath as an excellent way to "increase heart-rate variability and balance the stress-response system." In other words, this will activate our vagus nerve and bring us some peace and relaxation. With this practice each breath gets a little longer, but it should never feel uncomfortable. And if you feel at all dizzy, stop. Here are the steps:

1. Begin by getting comfortable, closing your eyes, and letting your body relax.
2. As you breathe in slowly, think, "In . . . two."
3. As you breathe out, think, "Out . . . two."
4. Repeat twice.
5. On your next breath in, think, "In . . . two . . . three" as you inhale.
6. Then think, "Out . . . two . . . three" as you exhale.
7. Repeat three times.
8. On your next breath in, think, "In . . . two . . . three . . . four" as you inhale.
9. Then think, "Out . . . two . . . three . . . four" as you exhale.
10. Repeat four times.[48]

Try doing this breath for five to ten minutes a day, once or twice a day. But do what works best for you.

Box Breathing

If you want to breathe like a Navy SEAL, this one is for you. The Navy SEALs use this technique to deal with the stress of their work. Also known as square breathing, this is a simple four-step technique you can do anywhere and anytime you're feeling stressed:

1. Begin by inhaling slowly to the count of four.
2. Hold your breath to the count of four.
3. Exhale to the count of four.
4. Hold to the count of four.

Then repeat until you feel calm.[49]

That's all there is to it, but breathing like this can really bring a sense of calm no matter how tense the situation.

Dr. Weil's 4-7-8 Relaxation Breath

Andrew Weil, MD, is a well-known pioneer in the field of integrative medicine, and his 4-7-8 relaxation breath exercise is recommended and used by people around the world. Not only is this a great way to ease anxiety, but Weil also recommends it for use before bed to help ease insomnia.

1. Begin by exhaling fully through your mouth with a whoosh.
2. Close your mouth and inhale quietly through your nose to the count of four.
3. Hold your breath and count to seven.
4. Exhale through your mouth with a whooshing sound to a count of eight.
5. Repeat the cycle four times.

Note: The inhale is done quietly, through your nose. The exhale is a whoosh through your mouth and is twice as long.[50]

The Rose and the Candle

I learned this last breath in a yoga class, and I've used it ever since. I love the simplicity and ease of it. This is easy to do and fun to imagine. Here are the steps:

1. Imagine you're holding a fragrant rose in one hand and a lit candle with a flickering flame in the other.
2. As you breathe in, lift that rose to your nose and imagine you're inhaling the beautiful scent of it. Breathe in deeply to enjoy the fragrance.
3. As you exhale, lower the rose and bring the glowing candle flame near your lips. Then gently and slowly blow on the flame until it flickers. You're not going to blow it out. You just want to make the flame dance a little.
4. Repeat until you feel calm.

You can do this breath anytime you're feeling anxious to restore a beautiful feeling of calm and peace.

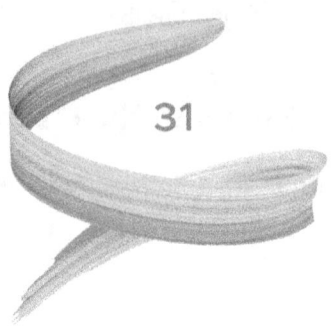

31

Meditation

From the earliest days, people have used meditation to focus their awareness in a way that helps bring a sense of calm to their bodies and their minds. And today we have a better understanding of how meditation works and how powerful it can be.

A 2022 study appearing in *JAMA* suggests that mindful meditation may work to calm anxiety as well as the commonly prescribed drug Lexapro (escitalopram).[51]

And, as Dr. Navaz Habib writes in his book *Activate Your Vagus Nerve*, "Heart rate variability studies have shown that meditation has significant positive benefits on vagus nerve function because as we meditate, our attention moves toward our breath."[52]

There's no doubt about it: meditation is a great way to ease anxiety. Maybe you already have a meditation practice in place and you're reaping the rewards. If so, keep up the good work.

But maybe you're like me. I've never really been able to get the hang of meditation. I sit, relax, and breathe, and almost immediately I start thinking about my to-do list and worrying that sitting there "doing nothing" is just wasting my time.

For most of my life, I've been a meditation dropout. And maybe that's true for you too. Maybe you believe that meditation is too complicated, demanding, or just plain weird for you.

Well, recently I've realized that meditation isn't some secret practice that only smarter, "better" people can master. Meditation is simply the act of listening to your breath and your body and letting go of everything else. That's all.

No complicated rules. No right way or wrong way. Nothing weird. Just listening. I don't know about you, but thinking about meditation that way makes it seem like something I can actually do.

And if meditation is nothing but a matter of listening, it seems to me that the trick to meditation is just a matter of learning how to be a good listener.

How to Listen

Listening in general is all about making a connection. When you listen to someone else, your intent is to connect with their thoughts and feelings. When you listen to the wind or the ocean, you connect with the world around you. And when you listen to your body and your mind, you connect with the truth about who you really are. Here are some things you can do to be a good listener and make those connections:

1. Slow down.
2. Be present. Be focused. Be compassionate.
3. Don't have an agenda. Listen with an open mind.
4. Be patient. Sometimes the best answers are the ones you have to wait for.
5. Don't try to fix anything. Listening isn't fixing or any other action.

That's all there is to it. Simple enough. But how do you get into a conversation with yourself?

The best way I know to do that is to use a technique I created that connects the body and the mind. I call it the *noticing breath*.

The Noticing Breath Meditation

All you have to do to connect body and mind is just start noticing your breath. Notice how cool the air is as you inhale and how warm the air is as you exhale. Maybe you can think or say "in" as you inhale and "out" as you exhale.

As you continue to notice your breath, let your body and your mind relax. And then just listen. If you do this even for just a few minutes, not only are your body and mind in communication—you're also meditating. It's that simple.

If this works for you, why not try to focus on your breath at a certain time every day? Maybe first thing in the morning or before bed. If this feels good and you want to explore a more formal kind of meditation practice, below are some other methods that just might work for you.

Guided Meditation

If meditation is a challenge for you, another great way to get started is to do a guided meditation. This is the practice of listening to someone else guide you through a meditation (or you can create your own guide). Again, all you have to do is relax and listen. You don't have to worry about focus or staying on track. Someone else does all that for you.

And not only is this a great way to get started, but it doesn't have to take long.

A 2019 study found that just thirteen minutes a day of listening to a guided meditation session for eight weeks "decreased negative mood state and enhanced attention, working memory and recognition memory as well as decreased anxiety state."[53]

That's all it takes. Just thirteen minutes a day.

But what if you're ready for a more traditional meditation practice?

Here's an age-old, time-tested technique that works even for me, the meditation dropout.

Mantra and Mudra—Kirtan Kriya Meditation

This technique is called Kirtan Kriya meditation.

Kirtan comes from Sanskrit and means *to sing* or refers to a song.

Kriya also comes from Sanskrit and means *to act*. And that's what this practice is: a combination of singing and taking action.

This practice comes from Kundalini yoga, but you don't have to go to a yoga class or sit in the lotus position to make this work. It's something you can do anytime you have a few minutes to spare.

And there's some real science that proves the power of this practice. A 2015 study in the *Journal of Alzheimer's Disease* found that the practice of Kirtan Kriya meditation can be helpful for people showing signs of cognitive distress. It "has also been shown to improve sleep, reduce depression, reduce anxiety, as well as offering a long list of spiritual, physical and psychological benefits."[54]

So, how does this work? All you need is a mantra and a mudra. Two things that sound complicated but are really simple.

Mantra

First of all, a mantra is just a word or phrase you repeat. And the mantra for this practice is as follows:

"Sa," "Ta," "Na," "Ma." Four syllables that represent our life cycle.

"Sa" is birth.

"Ta" is life.

"Na" is death.

"Ma" is rebirth.

And when we repeat them, we re-create our life cycle.

Birth. Life. Death. Rebirth.

Mudra

The mudra is simply the hand gesture that we make as we repeat the mantra. And if you have trouble sitting still, the nice thing about this meditation is that stillness isn't necessary. We get to move our hand and our mind in unison as we put the mantra and mudra together.

Practicing Kirtan Kriya

So, when you put the mantra and the mudra together, it looks like this:
  As you sing or say "Sa," touch your first finger to your thumb.
  As you sing or say "Ta," touch your middle finger to your thumb.
  As you sing or say "Na," touch your ring finger to your thumb.
  As you sing or say "Ma," touch your pinkie to your thumb.

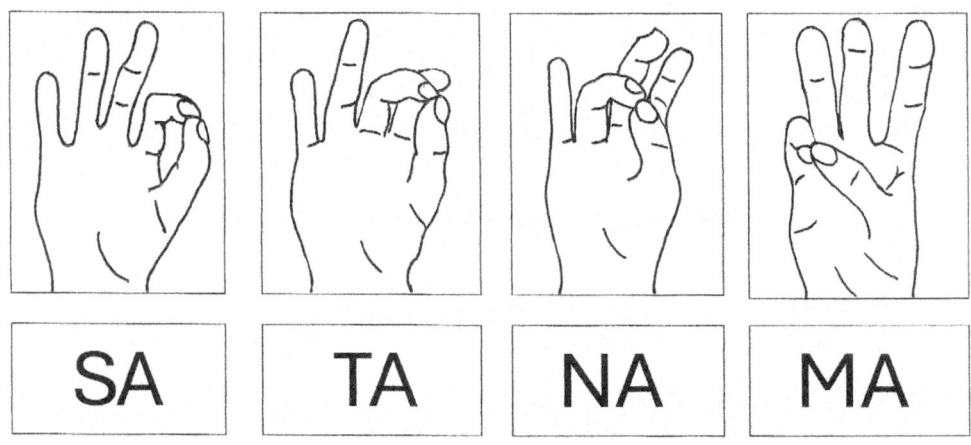

1. It's recommended that you begin by singing the syllables out loud a few times as you practice the mudra. Dharma Singh Khalsa's 2015 article in the *Journal of Alzheimer's Disease* suggests you sing the syllables to the first four notes of "Mary Had a Little Lamb," which works perfectly.[55]
2. Next, whisper those syllables out loud.
3. Then just think the syllables, again with the mudra.

When we say the syllables out loud, we're connecting to our physical body.

When we whisper them, we're connecting with our mind.

And when we just think them, we're connecting with our spirit.

So, it's body, mind, and spirit. And that's the entire practice.

For me, the best thing about this practice is that it's portable. If you don't want to sit and meditate, you can do this practice anywhere and anytime you feel the need to find some calm. Do it while you're in your doctor's waiting room, when you're stuck in traffic, or when you need to quiet your negative thoughts before bed.

Meditation Matters

No matter what kind of meditation you do, having a regular meditation practice can go a long way to creating the healthy, peaceful life you've always wanted.

It doesn't have to be complicated. You don't have to do it perfectly. You just have to listen.

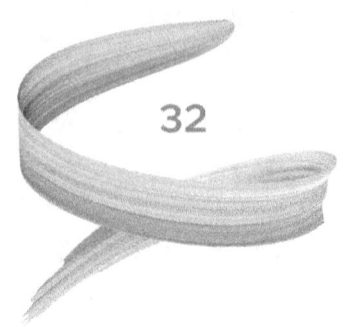

Acupressure

Acupuncture and acupressure are both ancient Chinese healing practices that work to improve circulation, reduce inflammation, balance our nervous system, and activate our vagus nerve.

They both involve pressing on various points located throughout the body to open blockages and stimulate our meridians—which I think of as highways of energy that connect various parts of our body. And, like traffic on a highway, when there's an obstruction or accident, the flow of that traffic has to be detoured, which then leads to tie-ups and confusion all the way down the line.

Both acupuncture and acupressure work the same way to clear those blockages and obstructions to get things running again. But with acupressure, you don't need needles to release that flow of energy. You can use your fingertips to get the same effect.

My favorite thing about acupressure is that you don't have to go to a professional to get all the physical and emotional benefits this practice has to offer. You can do it yourself. And you can use it anytime, anywhere, and in any anxiety-provoking situation.

It Works!

Before you write this practice off as some new age hokum, let me share that acupressure has been a real game changer for me. I use it throughout my day to help with digestion, clear my thinking, improve my circulation, and ease my anxiety.

A 2021 study published in *Complementary Therapies in Clinical Practice* even found that using acupuncture in conjunction with SSRIs (a widely used type of antidepressant) "can significantly improve anxiety state compared to anti-anxiety therapy using SSRIs alone."[56]

How to Do Acupressure

In my experience, everyone does acupressure a little differently. But in general, it's suggested that you begin your practice by locating the pressure point you want to use. Then apply steady, firm pressure with either your first two fingers or your thumb—whichever feels most comfortable for you. This should never hurt. It's recommended that you hold the point for two to three minutes.

As you massage the spot, breathe deeply and notice how relaxed you feel as your body connects with your brain and lets it know all is well and it can relax. Be on the lookout for a sigh, yawn, or swallow, all signs that your body is relaxing and sending that message of calm and peace to your brain.

But I do something a little different. The technique I use comes from qigong, and it works really well for me. Once I find the pressure point, I gently press on the point as I exhale and massage gently. As I inhale, I lift my fingers from the point. I pause, then press the point again with my next inhale. I think it works well for me because it keeps me focused on the pressure point and my breath at the same time. I repeat the practice until I experience a yawn or sigh, which let me know it's working.

There are over four hundred acupuncture points in our bodies. So, which ones are the best for easing anxiety?

Here are my five favorite anxiety-easing points:

1. **Yintang (Hall of Impressions) (EX-HN3)**

    This first point is located in the middle of your forehead in between your eyebrows. It is also known as your third eye. Many of us already use it instinctively to help us feel better. I often see people rubbing their foreheads when they're feeling frustrated or anxious, and for good reason.

    Some interesting research shows using this point can ease the anxiety of preoperative patients waiting to go into surgery.[57] And if it can ease anxiety in a high-stress situation like that, imagine what it will do for daily worries and fears.

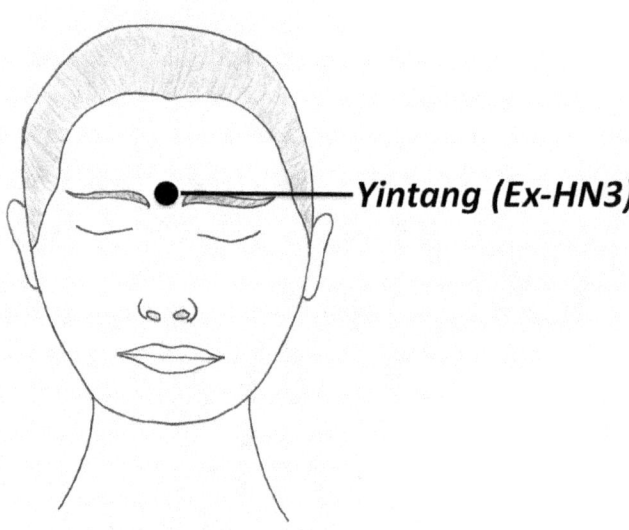

2. **Neiguan (Pericardium) (P6)**

To find this point, turn your palm up. Measure three finger widths down from the crease in your wrist. Then, with your thumb, find the valley between the two tendons in your wrist.

This powerful point is not only proven to slow your heartbeat and activate your vagus nerve, but it's also recommended by the Memorial Sloan Kettering Cancer Center (and me) to help with the nausea and vomiting that can come with chemotherapy or just life.[58]

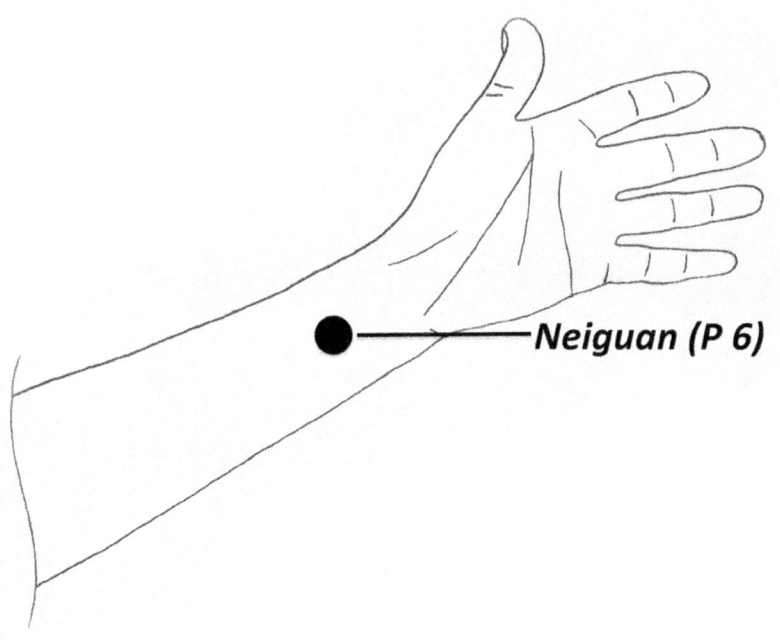

3. **Hegu (Union Valley) (LI 14)**

   This point is located between the thumb and the first finger, and I've heard it called the "Tylenol point" because it's supposed to work as well as Tylenol at relieving pain. In fact, Sloan Kettering recommends massaging this point to ease headaches, and I agree.[59]

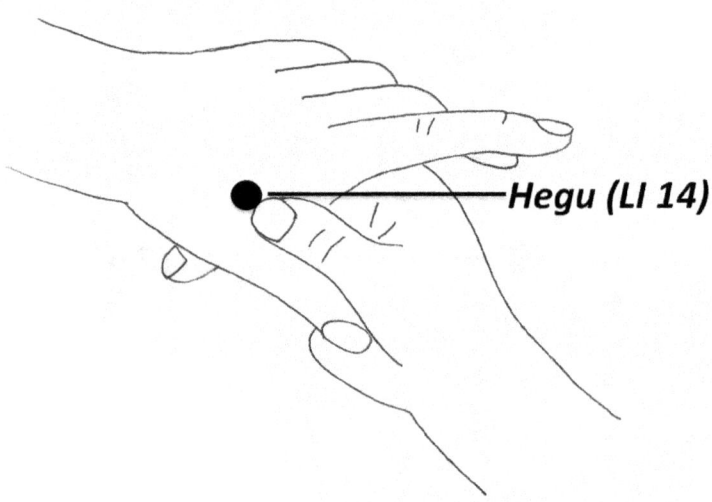

Acupressure

4. **Ear Shen Men (Spirit Gate, Gate of Life, Master Point)**

   This point is found in the upper third of the ear. To find it, rest your fingers on the top of your ear, then press your thumb into the indentation just below.[60]

   There are a number of really powerful acupressure points located in our ears (auricular points), but Ear Shen Men is known for creating a sense of calm and relaxation.

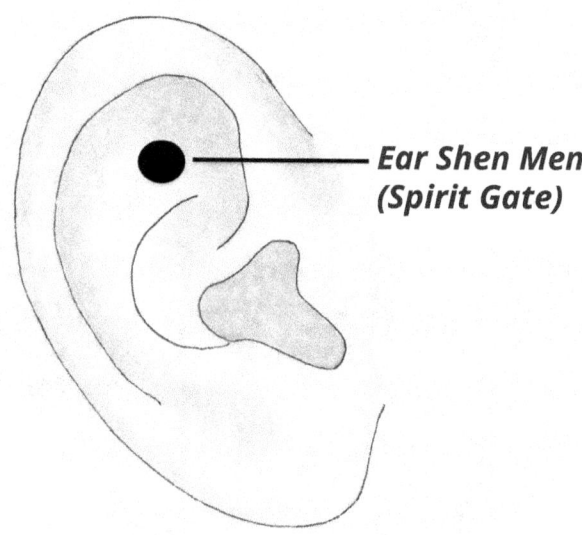

5. **Conception Vessel 17 (CV 14) (The Sea of Tranquility)**

    This anxiety-busting point is located in that indentation or dip in the center of your breastbone. You can press it in the usual way, or you can press your hands together in a prayer position, then press your thumbs against your breastbone at the level of your heart. Do whatever feels best for you.

    According to Michael Gach, PhD, author of *Acupressure for Emotional Healing*, when you're dealing with an anxiety attack, this point is "the single best point to use for relief."[61] I would agree that this point works to help slow my breathing and calm me when my anxiety or stress feels like it's going to get out of control.

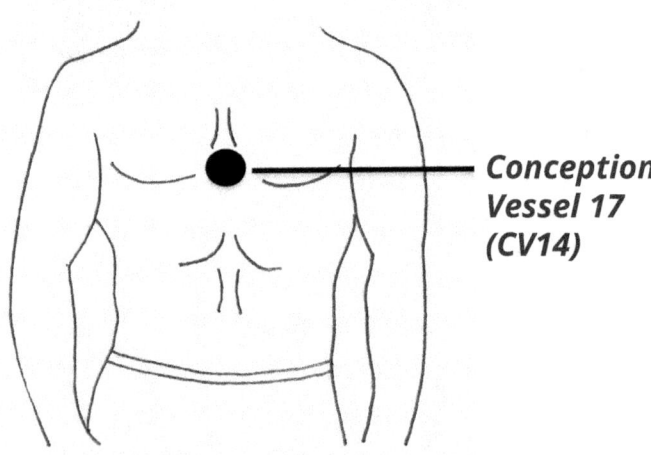

I use acupressure daily to help me relax, stay centered, and keep focused. I do it in response to any anxiety I'm feeling in the moment, and I do it as a regular practice to bring an ongoing sense of peace in my life.

I find as I massage these points, I can actually feel my body relax and my breath slow. And as I continue massaging and breathing, that sense of calm in my body creates the same sense of calm in my brain. I hope it works the same for you.

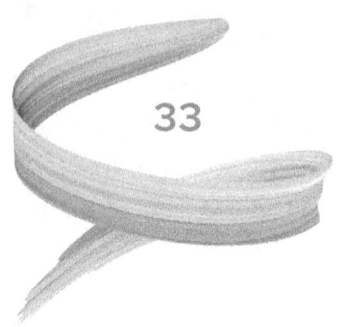

Massage

The Power of Touch

For at least five thousand years, humankind has been using massage to soothe pain, heal injuries, balance our bodies, and restore health.

Over the years there have been all sorts of massage methods and approaches. And while some may argue about which approach is best, what's clear is that human touch has the power to heal, both our body and our spirit. And today's research bears that out.

A study appearing in *Complementary Therapies in Clinical Practice* found that massage not only had physical benefits, but it also increased vagal activity, which served to reduce "anxiety, depression and heart rate."[62] So massage is not only good for the body; it's also good for the mind and the spirit.

According to the Mayo Clinic, an hour of massage lowers cortisol (the body's stress hormone) while increasing serotonin (the feel-good hormone). And that boosts "your body's ability to fight off pain, anxiety and feelings of sadness."[63]

So, you might want to go ahead and book yourself a massage. But here's some good news: you don't need a professional massage to get the benefits. You can do massage yourself, and you can even include self-massage as a part of your daily wellness plan.

DIY Massage Techniques to Ease Anxiety

While you probably can't do a full-body massage yourself, here are two techniques that are easy to do on your own and scientifically proven to work.

Shoulder Massage

A 2020 study in *Scientific Reports* found that not only did a shoulder massage reduce stress, but it increased relaxation, and it also increased vagal activity as well as activity in our PNS (peaceful nervous system).[64] No doubt about it, this one is simple to do, and it works. Here's how to give yourself a shoulder massage:

1. Place the palm of your right hand on your left shoulder.
2. Make gentle circles along your shoulder blade.
3. Work up the back of your neck.
4. Then work down to your upper left arm until you feel your shoulder relax.
5. Repeat on the other side.

Most of us can do this for ourselves. But if that's not possible, there are also head and neck massagers on the market that can be helpful. And of course, you can ask someone else to do that massage for you.

Foot Massage

Research also suggests that massaging your feet supports your general well-being (not to mention it feels great). And according to a 2010 study, foot reflexology (or massage) has been shown to increase vagal activity and decrease blood pressure.[65]

Best of all, a foot massage is something most of us can do ourselves.

Here's a technique that works for me:

1. Begin by sitting comfortably and, if possible, rest your right foot on your left thigh.
2. Take hold of your right foot with both hands. Then gently massage the top of your foot with your fingers, making small circles beginning at the ankle and working your way down to your toes and then back again. Repeat twice.
3. Continue to hold your foot with both hands, using them to gently rotate your foot. Repeat three times.
4. Gently stretch your toes toward you. Then, using the knuckles of your left hand, briskly rub the sole of your right foot to increase circulation and warm your foot. Repeat until your foot feels warm and you feel relaxed.
5. Repeat on the other side.

Alternate Foot Massage

If you're not able to do the foot massage described above, rolling a tennis ball back and forth and in circles on the ground with your bare foot can work just as well. I hope you'll give one or both of these techniques a try.

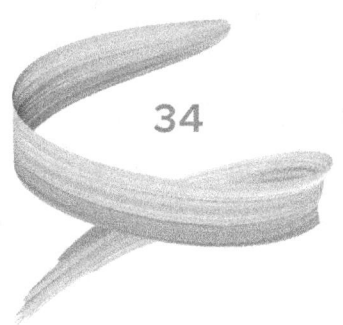

34

A Body in Motion

> **Warning:** As always, consult your health care provider to be sure these techniques are safe for you to try. And never, ever do anything that causes you pain. This is always about feeling better, never worse.

No doubt about it: exercise makes us stronger physically. It can also make us more agile and confident, and it may even help us live longer. But that's not all it can do. Exercise can also ease our anxiety.

A 2022 study of 286 adults found that people who exercised for just twelve weeks were less anxious and depressed than those who didn't.[66]

Even better, you don't have to run a marathon or climb a mountain to get the benefits of exercise. As Dr. Navaz Habib writes in *Activate Your Vagus Nerve*, "mild, low level exercise can stimulate the vagus nerve."[67]

But how much exercise do we need to get and stay healthy?

According to the *Physical Activity Guidelines for Americans*, issued by the U. S. Department of Health and Human Services, adults should get at least 150 to 300 minutes (2.5 hours to 5 hours) of moderate exercise activity a week. If we're enjoying more vigorous activity, we should get 75 to 150 minutes (1.25 hours to 2.5 hours) a week.[68]

So, now we know how much exercise we need to stay healthy. The next step is to get ourselves ready to move.

Finding the Fun

The first step to getting your body in gear is to find exercise that you enjoy. Join an exercise class, take a lesson, play with your children, clean your house, climb a mountain, dance along with your favorite YouTube video, or join a sports team. You can exercise indoors or out. You can work out alone or with others. No rules, no right, no wrong. Just what works for you.

It doesn't really matter what you do. What matters is that you do it. And if you love doing it, you're much more likely to keep showing up.

Here are some suggestions to get you off the couch.

An Alphabet of Active Fun:

- Aerobics
- Aikido
- Basketball
- Birding
- Boxing
- Canoeing
- Cleaning your house (or anything else you want)
- Dancing
- Elliptical machine
- Football
- Frisbee toss
- Gardening
- Golfing
- Hiking
- Isometrics
- Judo
- Jumping rope
- Karate
- Lacrosse
- Lunges
- Marching
- Mountain climbing
- Nordic walking
- Outdoor nature walking
- Paintball
- Pickleball
- Qigong
- Rock climbing
- Running
- Roller blading
- Skateboarding

- Skiing
- Shopping
- Swimming
- Trampolining
- Triathlon
- Unicycling
- Volleyball
- Walking
- X-training
- Yoga
- Zumba

So, what's one thing you've always loved doing or have been hoping to try?

Write it here: _____

_____

Now you've decided what you're going to do, the next step is to get ready to do it.

On Your Mark

Start by picking a goal that really inspires you, something you really want from exercise. Something that's going to make your life so much better. Imagine how it will look and feel to have it in your life. Visualize what your life would look like if you were stronger, more confident, and calmer. Having a goal that energizes you can get you up and moving.

Write that goal here: _____

_____

Get Set

The next step is to make sure you have everything you need for success. Having the right gear can make a real difference in how you feel about exercising. Make sure your shoes fit and that you have the right protective equipment and the right clothes. Create a great playlist of songs that inspire you.

Decide if and how you're going to keep track of your progress. Probably the best way to measure success is by how you feel, but lots of people find it motivating to count their steps, laps, or scores.

And finally decide exactly when you're going to start.

Write the day and time here: _____

_____

Now, go write that date and time on your calendar, enter it in your daily planner, or mark it wherever you keep track of your really important appointments. Because that's what this is. A Very Important Appointment. Which brings us to the last step.

Go!

Show up. No excuses. No whining. No compromising. Just show up and do it.

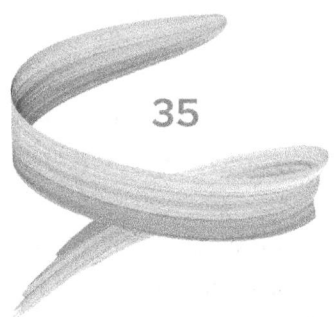

35

Splash Some Cold Water on It

Jump Right In

Here in New England, the social club known as the L Street Brownies is famous for celebrating every New Year by having members put on their bathing suits and plunge into the ice-cold waves of the Atlantic Ocean. I remember being a child and watching news clips of those "crazy guys" running into the ocean even when the thermometer registered temperatures near zero degrees.

Folks would shake their heads and say, "They have to be out of their minds."

But today's research proves exactly the opposite.

Today we know that running into ice-cold waves in January can have important health benefits. Immersing ourselves in cold water can help boost our immune system, ease stress, and reduce inflammation. Not only that, but research shows that exposure to cold stimulates the parasympathetic nervous system (peaceful nervous system), which can help bring a sense of calm.[69]

But if, like me, you don't want to plunge into ice-cold water to feel better physically, there are some easier, less dramatic things we can do.

> Important note: Jumping into the ocean or taking an ice-cold shower may not be the answer for everyone (at least not for me). And for some people it can be dangerous.
>
> According to the National Center for Cold Water Safety, "Plunging into frigid water is stressful on the body and can have harmful effects. Hypothermia, mainly. And in rare cases immersion can provoke cardiac arrest, arrhythmia or respiratory distress, particularly in people with underlying health issues."[70]

Icing the Vagus Nerve

There's been a lot of talk about vagus nerve icing on TikTok. Lots of people have reported trying it, but is this just an internet fad, or does it work?

It turns out that it works.

A 2018 study found that cold stimulation applied to the neck, cheek, and right forearm for just sixteen seconds slowed heart rates.[71] So, if you're ready to ice your vagus nerve, grab a cold compress or put a few ice cubes in a plastic baggie and gently press it against your neck or cheek. Or you can end your shower with a blast of cold water on the back of your neck.

Splash Cold Water on Your Face

This one works for me. And I'm so glad I don't have to take a polar plunge or a freezing shower to get the benefits of cold water. It turns out that splashing cold water on your face also works to relax the body and the mind. In fact, I often just wipe my face and neck with a cold, wet facecloth, and that seems to work well.

Drink a Glass of Ice-Cold Water

This is the easiest way of all to include cold water in your life. A study done in 2010 found that drinking a glass of ice-cold water can activate the vagus nerve and at the same time slow our heart rate.[72] Best of all, adding an icy drink to your day is something most of us can do. No muss, no fuss.

Some or all of these techniques might not be right for you. I hope you'll listen to your body and do what feels good. And if you have any preexisting health conditions, please check in with your health care provider before taking the plunge.

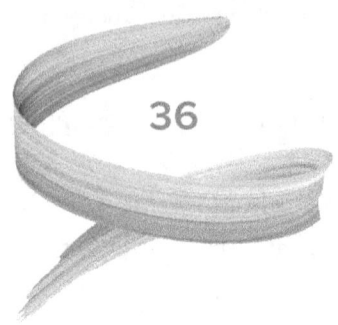

36

Music

Sing

Do you sing in the shower? Do you turn up the music and sing along when you're alone in your car? Or maybe you shine at karaoke?

Good for you. Not only are you expressing yourself, but you may also be lowering your blood pressure, improving your mood, easing stress, and stimulating your vagus nerve, all at the same time. A 2020 article in *Psychology Today* explains, "The vagus nerve connects to your vocal cords, making sounds stimulates the nerve and increases our heart-rate variability and vagal tone."[73] In other words, that connection is why singing can bring us a sense of calm and ease.

Sing with Others

But you don't have to go it alone. And there can be some added benefits from getting together and singing with a group. Singing with others can strengthen our sense of social connections and your relationships in a way that brings energy to our spirit and our vagus nerve.[74]

Humming and Chanting

It's not just singing that activates the vagus nerve. Research shows that chanting and humming work just as well, and sometimes better. It's that long, slow exhale that causes your PNS to kick in and your body to relax.[75]

It doesn't matter whether you chant as part of your yoga practice, hum quietly as you make your breakfast, or grab the mic at your local gathering place and belt out a song at the top of your lungs. It's the act of making sound that activates our vagus nerve.

Listen Up

But we don't have to sing, chant, or hum to use music to stimulate the vagus nerve. We can just sit back and listen to the music we love. And now we have some understanding about how listening to music works to bring us a sense of calm.

According to a 2022 study, "The vagus nerve, cranial nerve X, is located near the eardrum and responds to musical vibrations by triggering the body to relax." And while the study focused on listening to classical music, it found that fast music uplifted the listeners, slow music calmed them, and everyone felt better.[76]

No doubt about it: music helps ease anxiety. And whether you sing, hum, chant, or just listen, music can play an important role in activating your vagus nerve and bringing a sense of calm into your life.

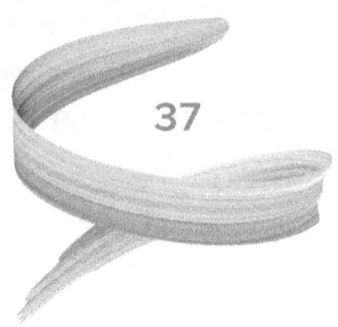

37

Laughter

Laughter is medicine for the body, the soul, and the vagus nerve. Any movement of our diaphragm activates our vagus nerve. And hearty laughter is a powerful way to get our diaphragm in motion. As Dr. Navaz Habib writes in *Activate Your Vagus Nerve*, laughter is like "exercise for the vagus nerve."[77]

And best of all, we can use laughter on purpose. That means we can use it anytime we want to interrupt our loops of negative thinking or to ease tension in our body.

Not to mention the fact that laughter is fun, it brightens our day, and it helps us connect with the people around us.

Now, maybe you don't think you have much of a sense of humor, or you don't feel much like laughing these days. Not to worry. There are ways to make laughter a part of your life, no matter who you are. Humor isn't something you have or you don't have. It's not some mystical process or something that happens by chance. Like so many things, humor can be learned, and you get better by practicing it. The trick here is to embrace the process and start small.

If a belly laugh is out of the question right now, no worries. You can start with a smile, which is easier and just as effective.

And you can keep that good feeling going by smiling throughout the day as often as possible. Because when you share your smile with the people around you, they may smile back. Our smiles connect us with the people around us without having to say a word. It's a universal language we can always use, even during the isolation of a pandemic, even with people you see at a distance. You never know what a gift your smile could be to someone who's going through a hard time.

So, start with a smile.

But laughter is a smile with a megaphone. It can boost your mood and your immune system. It can ease tension and, best of all, soothe anxiety. And the more you laugh, the better.

What Makes *You* Laugh?

What books, movies, TV shows, or YouTube videos crack you up? Is there a comedian who makes you laugh out loud? Do you have a friend who knows how to tell a joke? Is there a memory that makes you chuckle? How about spending time with puppies or kittens or going to a funny movie?

Whatever it is that makes you laugh, including more of it in your life is a great way to feel better and calmer both physically and emotionally.

How to Make Yourself Laugh

So far, we've been talking about spontaneous laughter, or laughter that's our reaction to an external event. Someone tells a joke and we laugh. But there's another kind of laughter, called simulated laughter, which we can choose to do. It's not our reaction to anything funny; it's something we simply choose to do.

Here's what's interesting. According to Ramon Mora-Ripoll, MD, "The body cannot distinguish between simulated and spontaneous laughter; therefore, their corresponding health effects are alleged to be alike." In other words, fake laughing has the same beneficial effects as a spontaneous belly laugh.

Here are some techniques taken from Mora-Ripoll's article "Simulated Laughter Techniques for Therapeutic Use in Mental Health." You can use them to get yourself laughing, no matter what.

Laugh Out Loud

1. **Laugh with the vowels.** This is a great technique to use if you're having trouble getting started. Simply wave your arms in the air and laugh all the vowels out loud.

    "Ha, ha, ha. He, he, he. Hi, hi, hi. Ho, ho, ho. Hu, hu, hu." Repeat as long as it feels good.

2. **Laugh like a lion.** Stand in front of a mirror and look yourself in the eye. Open your mouth as wide as possible. Stick out your tongue. Wave your paws in the air and laugh-roar like a lion.

3. **Laugh with your whole body.** Laugh while you make faces, flap your arms, hop on one foot, wiggle, stretch, twist, or move in any way that feels like fun.[78]

Laugh It Off

And whenever you can, laugh with yourself. Imagine what it would look like if we could go through life knowing we could always laugh away our mistakes. I love this idea. I'm thinking it would be like having a big pink eraser you can use on any errors you've made. Wouldn't that make things so much easier? Knowing you wouldn't have to be perfect and you would still be okay? Laughter gives you that power. It's a big pink eraser that can set you free from the need to be perfect. Just laugh it off.

Part Five

Creating Your Personalized Plan for Healing Your Anxiety

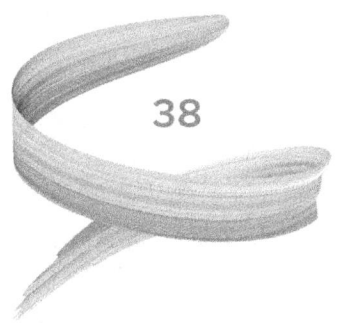

Find Out What's Really Causing Your Anxiety
The Quiz

We're all starting our healing journey from different places. Maybe you're dealing with pain and trauma from childhood or a catastrophic life event. Maybe you're overwhelmed by constant thoughts of terrible things that could happen in the future, or maybe you have a physical condition that causes stress or tension in your body.

So, the first step in healing your anxiety is to figure out exactly what your anxiety looks like today. And to do that, you just need to take this quick and easy anxiety self-assessment.

Don't worry—there are no right or wrong answers here. Just the truth about the role anxiety is playing in your life.

As you answer the questions, I suggest you be on the lookout for clues about all the ways that anxiety is impacting your life. Maybe you'll recognize an unexpected pattern of negative thinking, or you'll spot a deeply held self-doubt that's holding you back. Maybe you'll see that your anxiety has more than one cause, the source of your anxiety has changed, or that your anxiety is having more of an impact on you than you'd realized.

Anxiety Self-Assessment

Circle all the statements below that best apply to you:

1. I'm afraid that if people knew the truth about me, they wouldn't like me.
2. Things might be going well now, but I know something awful is about to happen.
3. I have trouble sleeping.

1. I'm afraid to speak up for myself. What if I say something wrong or stupid?
2. I'm not safe. The world is not safe.
3. I have unexplained headaches.

1. I'm afraid of conflict. I'm afraid of my own anger. I'm afraid of making someone else angry at me.
2. I can't trust people. I can't count on anyone.
3. I tremble or shake.

1. I'm afraid everything won't be perfect. I'm afraid my work isn't good enough.
2. I spend time imagining possible future disasters and catastrophes.
3. I have unexplained shortness of breath. I sometimes feel like I'm suffocating.

1. I'm afraid people will find out the shameful things I've done in the past.
2. I believe imagining the worst will protect me from or prepare me for any possible disaster.
3. I have unexplained chest pains.

Find Out What's Really Causing Your Anxiety

1. I'm afraid of losing control.
2. I worry I'm going to lose everything, and I'll end up homeless.
3. I'm restless and have trouble concentrating.

1. I'm afraid I'm not capable of taking care of myself, so I work hard at pleasing others so they'll take care of me.
2. I worry constantly about my health and the health of people around me.
3. I have unexplained digestive distress.

1. I don't deserve a good life. I don't deserve to succeed. I don't deserve to have what I want.
2. I worry I won't be able to protect myself and those I love from harm.
3. I have chills or sweats.

1. I'm not smart enough. I'm not capable. I'm not good at anything.
2. I worry about climate change, world hunger, natural disasters, and war.
3. I have unexplained dizziness or sense of weakness.

1. I'm afraid I'm not loveable. No one could ever really love me.
2. I worry that I'm going to die alone.
3. I grit my teeth or clench my jaw.

Let's Look at the Numbers

_____ How many number 1 answers did you circle? (Self-doubt)

_____ How many number 2 answers did you circle? (Fear of change)

_____ How many number 3 answers did you circle? (Physical anxiety)

Now, put them in order.

_____ The number you circled the most.

_____ The number you circled next.

_____ The number you circled the least.

> If you circled **number 1** the most,
> chances are you're dealing with self-doubt.
>
> If you circled **number 2** the most,
> chances are you're dealing with fear of change.
>
> If you circled **number 3** the most,
> chances are you're dealing with physical anxiety.

Now that you've spent some time getting to know specifics about your anxiety, the next step is to put together a plan of action that works for you. And here's how to do that.

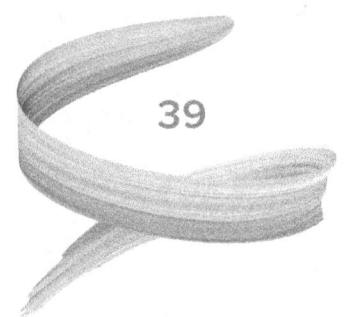

Getting Started

Self-Doubt

If you circled the number 1 questions most, chances are the traumas and negative beliefs from your past are making you anxious.

Self-doubt is lack of faith in your ability to handle what's going to happen in your life. It's the result of all that baggage we're dragging around from our past. It's all those things you keep telling yourself about what you can't do. It's an echo of all the things people in your past have told you about your limitations and shortcomings. It's the story you tell yourself about all the times you failed, messed up, were embarrassed, or felt guilty or ashamed.

Self-doubt is that voice in your head that tells you over and over you're not good enough.

To start feeling better right now, turn to the section on self-doubt and find one or two things you think might work for you.

Write them here: _____

_____

_____

Fear of Change

If you circled the number 2 questions most, your worried thoughts about the future may be causing your anxiety.

Fear of change involves worrying about the future. The fact is that the only thing in life we can count on is change, and there's nothing we can do about that. We have no control over what's going to happen to us in the future. Fear of change isn't really about what might happen in the future; it's about what we *think* might happen to us.

To get started on feeling better right now, head to the section on fear of change and find one or two things you think might work for you.

Write them here: _____

_____

Physical Anxiety

If you circled the number 3 questions most, what's going on in your body might be making you anxious.

Our body and our mind are connected and in constant communication with each other. Recent research proves that the stress and tension in our body can have a real effect on what we think. The fear in our body can cause anxiety in our brain.

To get started on feeling better right now, turn to the section on physical anxiety and find one or two things you think might work for you.

Write them here: _____

_____

If you circled the same number of answers in two categories, start with the section that feels right to you. Maybe there was one question that stuck out to you as important, or maybe there was something you hadn't thought about before and would like to learn more about. Start there.

Once you've turned to the section you've chosen, read through it. Try all the exercises, or just do the ones that appeal to you. This is your book. This is your equation, and your solution is going to be uniquely yours.

If something doesn't work for you the first time, I recommend trying it again later. And if something stops working for you, stop doing it. As you continue to try new ideas and approaches, imagine that you're putting together a tool kit of ways you can ease your anxiety no matter what the circumstances.

Again, there are no right or wrong answers here. Just the answers that work for you!

Know What You Want and Set a "Go Get It" Goal

Now that you're on your way to creating a calmer life, it's important to stay on track and keep moving and motivated. The best way I know to do that is to set a clear goal for what you want.

So, let me ask you: What is it you want?

Write your goal here: _____

_____

All right, that's a good start. But a simple goal may not be enough to inspire you to take action. What we need is an extraordinary goal—one that gets you out of bed and keeps you going, even through the darkest days. We need a goal that makes us shiver with excitement and sets our imagination on fire. And to uncover that, let's take a deeper dive into what your life is going to look like when you have what you really want.

Why I Want What I Want

Write your answers to the following questions:

1. What will reaching my goal look like in my life? _____
   _____

2. What will reaching it feel like? _____
   _____

3. Reaching this goal means I'll be able to: _____
   _____

4. Reaching this goal means I'll be able to help: _____
   _____

5. Reaching this goal means I'll never have to: _____
   _____

6. I know reaching this goal is possible because I can depend on:
   _____
   _____

7. The best thing about reaching my goal will be: _____
   _____

I hope as you answer these questions, you get excited by the possibilities that lie ahead for you. Let your imagination go wild. Have fun with this. For a change, start imagining the very best, and let that inspire you to take the next step and the step after that.

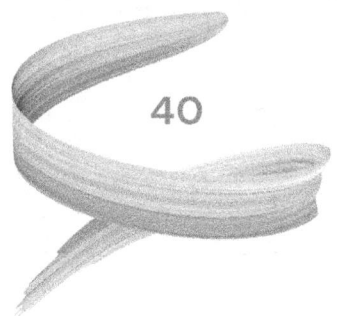

40

Staying on Track

Finally, it's important to stay on course throughout your healing journey. And to do that, I recommend you track your progress.

I suggest you come back here at least once a week and repeat the three steps at the end of this chapter. Figure out where you are. Remind yourself why it matters. Then decide what tools and techniques you want to use for the week. You can keep track on your Weekly Success Planner that follows or in any other way that works for you. Keeping track not only requires you to focus on these important questions, but it also gives you a complete record of what worked for you and what didn't.

When you get stuck, you can come back to your weekly planner and remind yourself of the times when things went right. Work to repeat that success. Looking back can also remind you of how far you've come, and it can help you avoid whatever caused you to go off course.

My Weekly Success Planner

This week my anxiety is showing up like this: _____

_____

_____

_____

The techniques I'm choosing to use are: _____

_____

_____

_____

This week I will: _____

_____

_____

_____

_____

Success matters to me because: _____

_____

_____

_____

I know I can do this because: _____

_____

_____

_____

Uh-Oh!

Like everything else in life, the path to finding peace is never smooth. You're going to run into tough days, hard times, detours, delays, and complete catastrophes. You're going to get lost and anxious, and there are going to be days or weeks when you just give up. That's to be expected. It's all part of life.

But just because you've stopped a while doesn't mean you're giving up for good.

Here's the truth about life that successful people have learned: It doesn't matter how many times you've fallen down. What matters is that you get back up and try again and again until you have what you want.

And that means no matter what you've been through, no matter how tough the circumstance, no matter how long it's been since you were on track—you can start in this moment. Take one tiny, tiny step toward feeling better.

To do that, all you have to do is come back to these three simple steps:

1. Take the assessment.
2. Remind yourself of how it's going to feel to achieve that goal of yours.
3. Pick the methods that feel right for you today, and maybe do just one thing. Walk to the mailbox. Call a friend. Watch a funny video. Maybe you want to do what's worked for you in the past, or you might want to try something new. Just do something. That's the secret. I know from personal experience that action of any kind is the world's best antidote for anxiety. Go get busy.

That's all there is to it. To start, to start over, to reclaim your life, to begin your healing journey, all you have to do is take those three simple steps.

And the good news is that anytime you're struggling, you can come back here and start over. You can do these three steps every morning, once a month, or you can adapt them any way you'd like to suit yourself and your lifestyle.

If someone in your life is struggling with anxiety, you can also share these steps and encourage them to create their own plan.

Because we're all in this together, and we've got this!

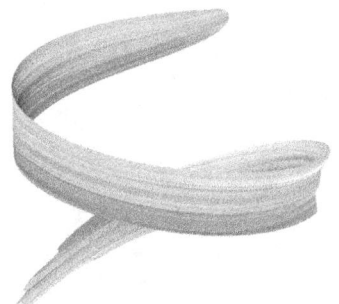

Conclusion: The Journey Ahead

It's an honor and joy to be a part of your healing journey. But it doesn't have to end here. You can continue to use this book as a guide, a support system, and a place to find encouragement anytime you'd like.

You can take the anxiety self-assessment quiz as often as you'd like to put together a new plan for your unique healing needs. And you can fill out your weekly success tracker as often as you'd like to keep yourself motivated.

If you're looking for some extra support, please join me at WendyLeeds.com or listen to my podcast, *Anxiety Connection*.

Let's not do this alone anymore.

Please keep in touch.

Warmly,
Wendy

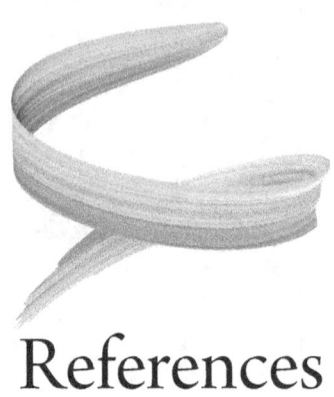

References

1. "Evolutionary Psychology," *Psychology Today*, 2019, https://www.psychologytoday.com/us/basics/evolutionary-psychology.

2. Rick Hanson, "Overcoming the Negativity Bias," *Dr. Rick Hanson* (blog), accessed April 26, 2024, https://www.rickhanson.net/overcoming-negativity-bias/.

3. Donald Hebb, *The Organization of Behavior* (Wiley, 1949).

4. Brian Hsueh et al., "Cardiogenic Control of Affective Behavioral State," *Nature* 615, no. 7951, (March 1, 2023): 292–299, https://doi.org/10.1038/s41586-023-05748-8.

5. Rolf Kleber, "Trauma and Public Mental Health: A Focused Review," *Frontiers in Psychiatry* 25, no. 10 (June 2019): 451, https://doi.org/10.3389/fpsyt.2019.00451.

6. Bessel Van Der Kolk, MD. *The Body Keeps the Score: Brain, Mind, and Body in the Healing of Trauma* (Penguin Books, 2014), 205.

7. Rhonda Britten, *Fearless Living: Live Without Excuses and Love Without Regret* (Berkeley Publishing, 2001), 67–79.

8. Lisa Firestone, PhD, "Why Many People Can't See Themselves Positively," *Psychology Today*, August 18, 2021, https://www.psychologytoday.com/us/blog/compassion-matters/202108/why-many-people-cant-see-themselves-positively.

9. Susan Jeffers, *Feel the Fear . . . And Do It Anyway* (Random House, 1987).

10. "Forgiveness: Your Health Depends on It," Hopkins Medicine, accessed April 22, 2024, https://www.hopkinsmedicine.org/health/wellness-and-prevention/forgiveness-your-health-depends-on-it.

11. "Forgiveness," American Psychological Association, accessed April 22, 2024, https://www.apa.org/topics/forgiveness.

12 Carissa Wilkes, Rob Kidd, Mark Sagar, and Elizabeth Broadbent, "Upright Posture Improves Affect and Fatigue in People with Depressive Symptoms," *Journal of Behavior Therapy and Experimental Psychiatry* 54 (March 2017): 143–149, https://doi.org/10.1016/j.jbtep.2016.07.015.

13 Fernado Marmolejo-Ramos et al., "Your Face and Moves Seem Happier When I Smile," *Journal of Experimental Psychology* 67, no. 1 (January 14, 2022): 14–22, https://doi.org/10.1027/1618-3169/a000470.

14 Adam Hajo and Adam D. Galinsky, "Enclothed Cognition," *Journal of Experimental Social Psychology* 48, no. 4 (July 2012): 918–925, https://doi.org/10.1016/j.jesp.2012.02.008.

15 Archy O. Berker et al., "Computations of Uncertainty Mediate Acute Stress Responses in Humans," *Nature Communications* 7 (March 29, 2016), https://doi.org/10.1038/ncomms10996.

16 Bill St. John, "Kitchen Mistakes: Toll House Cookies, Potato Chips & Popsicles Were All Mistakes," UC Health, July 27, 2021, https://www.uchealth.org/today/kitchen-mistakes-toll-house-cookies-potato-chips-and-popsicles/.

17 Alyson Krueger, "15 Life-Changing Inventions That Were Created by Mistake," *Business Insider*, November 16, 2010, https://www.businessinsider.com/these-10-inventions-were-made-by-mistake-2010-11?op=1.

18 "Mt. Major: A Family-Friendly Hike with Fanatic-Friendly Views," *NH State Parks* (blog), June 28, 2016, https://blog.nhstateparks.org/mt-major-family-friendly-hike/.

19 Christopher Cascio et al., "Self-Affirmation Activates Brain Systems Associated with Self-Related Processing and Reward and is Reinforced by Future Orientation," *Social Cognition and Affective Neuroscience* 11, no. 4 (April 11, 2014): 621–629, https://doi.org/10.1093/scan/nsv136.

20 Darby E. Saxbe and Rena Repetti, "No Place Like Home: Home Tours Correlate with Daily Patterns of Mood and Cortisol," *Personality and Social Psychology Bulletin* 36, no. 1 (January 2010): 71–81, https://doi.org/10.1177/0146167209352864.

21 Rene Marois and Jason Ivanoff, "Capacity Limits of Information Processing in the Brain," *Trends in Cognitive Sciences* 9, no. 6, (June 2005): 296–305, https://doi.org/10.1016/j.tics.2005.04.010.

22 Libby Sander, PhD, "Marie Kondo Tidying Up: This Is What Clutter Does to Your Body and Brain," *Newsweek*, January 22, 2019, https://www.newsweek.com/tidying-marie-kondo-clutter-netflix-life-changing-magic-tidying-mental-health-1299938.

23 Cheng Xu and Wenhua Yan, "The Relationship Between Information Overload and State of Anxiety in the Period of Regular Epidemic Prevention and Control in China: A Moderated Multiple Mediation Model," *Current Psychology* (June 6, 2022): 1–18, https://doi.org/10.1007/s12144-022-03289-3.

24 Nikki Puccetti et al., "Linking Amygdala Persistence to Real-World Emotional Experience and Psychological Well-Being," *Journal of Neuroscience* 41, no. 16 (September 2023): 3721–3730, https://doi.org/10.1523/JNeurosci.1637-20.2021.

25 Gaeton Chevalier, "The Effect of Grounding the Human Body on Mood," *Psychological Report* 116, no. 2 (April 2015): 534–542, https://doi.org/10.2466/06.PR0.116k21w5.

26 Cameron Anderson, Dacher Keltner, and Oliver P. John, "Emotional Convergence Between People Over Time," *Journal of Personality and Social Psychology* 84, no. 5 (May 2003): 1054–1068, https://doi.org/10.1037/0022-3514.84.5.1054.

27 Ellen Vora, MD, *The Anatomy of Anxiety: Understanding and Overcoming the Body's Fear Response* (HarperCollins, 2022), 169.

28 Vora, *Anatomy of Anxiety*, 24.

29 "The Brain-Gut Connection," Hopkins Medicine, accessed April 23, 2024, https://www.hopkinsmedicine.org/health/wellness-and-prevention/the-brain-gut-connection.

30 Suhrid Banskota, Jean-Eric Ghia, and Waliul Khan, "Serotonin in the Gut: Blessing or a Curse," *Biochimie* 161 (June 2019): 56–64, https://doi.org/10.1016/j.biochi.2018.06.008.

31 Stephen W. Porges, "The Biological Psychology," *Biological Psychology Journal* 74, no. 2, (February 2007): 117–143, https://doi.org/10.1016/j.biopsycho.2006.06.009.

32 Stanley Rosenberg, *Accessing the Healing Power of the Vagus Nerve: Self-Help Exercises for Anxiety, Depression, Trauma, and Autism* (North Atlantic Books, 2017), 30.

33 Rosenberg, *Accessing the Healing Power*, 187–194, 208–210.

34 "Anxiety Disorders," Mayo Clinic, May 4, 2018, https://www.mayoclinic.org/diseases-conditions/anxiety/symptoms-causes/syc-20350961/2012/809653.

35 Rachel Reiff Ellis, "What Meds Might Cause Anxiety," WebMD, February 26, 2024, https://www.webmd.com/anxiety-panic/anxiety-causing-meds.

References

36 Michael B. Gottschalk, PhD, and Katarina Domschke, MD, PhD, "Genetics of Generalized Anxiety Disorder and Related Traits," *Dialogues in Clinical Neuroscience* 19, no. 2 (June 2017): 159–168, https://doi.org/10.31887/DCNS.2017.19.2/kdomschke.

37 Nicole van Beek and Eric Griez, "Anxiety Sensitivity in First-Degree Relatives of Patients with Panic Disorder," *Behavioral Research and Therapy* 4, no. 8 (August 2003): 949–957, https://doi.org/10.1016/S0005-7967(02)00129-8.

38 Madison C. Piotrowski, MD, Julia Lunsford, and Bradley N. Gayes, MD, MPH, "Lifestyle Psychiatry for Depression and Anxiety: Beyond Diet and Exercise," *Lifestyle Medicine* 2, no. 1 (January 15, 2021), https://doi.org/10.1002/lim2.21.

39 Paul Thagard and Brandon Aubie, "Emotional Consciousness: A Neural Model of How Cognitive Appraisal and Some Somatic Perception Interact to Produce Qualitative Experience," Consciousness & Cognition 17, no. 3 (October 2008): 811–834, https://doi.org/10.1016/j.concog.2007.05.014.

40 "Stress Effects on the Body," APA, updated March 8, 2023, https://www.apa.org/topics/stress/body.

41 Dan Witters and Sangeeta Agrawl, "The Economic Cost of Poor Employee Mental Health," Gallup, updated December 2022, https://www.gallup.com/workplace/404174/economic-cost-poor-employee-mental-health.aspx.

42 "Anxiety Sensitivity," *Health Harvard*, March 9, 2014, https://www.health.harvard.edu/newsletter_article/Anxiety_sensitivity.

43 Andrea Zaccaro et al., "How Breath-Control Can Change Your Life: A Systematic Review on Psycho-Physiological Correlates of Slow Breathing," *Frontiers in Human Neuroscience* 12 (September 7, 2018): 353, https://doi.org/10.3389/fnhum.2018.00353.

44 Marc A. Russo, Danielle M Santarelli, and Dean O'Rourke, "The Physiological Effects of Slow Breathing in the Healthy Human," *Breathe* 13, no. 4 (December 2017): 298–309, https://doi.org/10.1183/20734735.009817.

45 Marjke DeCouck et al., "How Breathing Can Help You Make Better Decisions: Two Studies on the Effects of Breathing Patterns on Heart Rate Variability and Decision-Making in Business Cases," *International Journal of Psychophysiology* 139 (May 2019): 1–9, https://doi.org/10.1016/j.ijpsycho.2019.02.011.

46 Shu-Zhen Wang et al., "Effect of Slow Abdominal Breathing Combined with Biofeedback on Blood Pressure and Heart Rate Variability in

Prehypertension," *Journal of Complementary Medicine* 16, no. 10 (October 2010): 1039–1045, https://doi.org/10.1089/acm.2009.0577.

47 Roderik J. S. Gerritsen and Guido P. H. Band, "Breath of Life: The Respiratory Vagal Stimulation Model of Contemplative Activity," *Frontiers in Human Neuroscience* 12 (October 9, 2018): 397, https://doi.org/10.3389/fnhum.2018.00397.

48 Richard P. Grown, MD, and Patricia L. Gerbarg, MD, *The Healing Power of the Breath: Simple Techniques to Reduce Stress and Anxiety, Enhance Concentration and Balance Your Emotions* (Shambala Publications, 2012).

49 Karthnik Kumar, MBBS, "Why Do Navy SEALs Use Box Breathing?" *MedicineNet*, November 2021, https://www.medicinenet.com/why_do_navy_seals_use_box_breathing/article.htm.

50 Andrew Weil, MD, "The Art and Science of Breathing," Dr. Weil, accessed April 25, 2024, https://www.drweil.com/health-wellness/balanced-living/meditation-inspiration/the-art-and-science-of-breathing/.

51 Elizabeth A. Hoge, "Mindfulness-Based Stress Reduction vs Escitalopram for the Treatment of Adults with Anxiety Disorders: A Randomized Clinical Trial," *JAMA Psychiatry* 80, no. 1 (January 1, 2023): 13–21, https://doi.org/10.1001/jamapsychiatry.2022.3679.

52 Navaz Habib, *Activate Your Vagus Nerve: Unleash Your Body's Natural Ability to Heal* (Ulysses Press, 2019), 149–150.

53 Julia, C. Basso et al., "Brief, Daily Meditation Enhances Attention, Memory, Mood, and Emotional Regulation in Non-Experienced Meditators," *Behavioral Brain Research* 356 (January 2019): 208–220, https://doi.org/10.1016/j.bbr.2018.08.023.

54 Dharma Singh Khalsa, "Stress, Meditation, and Alzheimer's Disease Prevention: Where the Evidence Stands," *Journal of Alzheimer's Disease* 48, no. 1 (August 28, 2015): 1–12, https://doi.org/10.3233/JAD-142766.

55 Khalsa, "Stress, Meditation, and Alzheimer's Disease."

56 Ali Sabbagh Gol et al., "Additive Effects of Acupuncture in Alleviating Anxiety: A Double-Blind, Three-Arm, Randomized Clinical Trial," *Complementary Theories in Clinical Practices* 45 (August 4, 2021): 101466, https://doi.org/10.1016/j.ctcp.2021.101466.

57 Chan-Young Kwon, KMD, and Boram Lee, MD, "Acupuncture or Acupressure on *Yintang* (EX-HN3) for Anxiety: A Preliminary Review," *Medical Acupuncture* 30, no. 2 (April 1, 2018): 73–79, https://doi.org/10.1089/acu.2017.1268.

References

58 "Acupressure for Nausea and Vomiting," MSKCC, June 2022, https://www.mskcc.org/cancer-care/patient-education/acupressure-nausea-and-vomiting.

59 "Acupressure for Pain and Headaches," MSKCC, March 2023, https://www.mskcc.org/cancer-care/patient-education/acupressure-pain-and-headaches.

60 Yong-Chang P. Arai et al., "Auricular Acupuncture at the 'Shenmen' and 'Point Zero' Points Induced Parasympathetic Activation," *Evidence-Based Complementary Alternative Medicine* 945063 (June 4, 2013): https://doi.org/10.1155/2013/945063.

61 Michael Reed Gach, PhD, and Beth Ann Henning, Dipl, ABT, *Acupressure for Emotional Healing: A Self-Care Guide for Trauma, Stress & Common Emotion Imbalances* (Bantam Books, 2004), 89.

62 Tiffany Field, "Massage Therapy Research Review," *Complementary Therapies in Clinical Practices* 20, no. 4 (August 1, 2014): 224–229, https://doi.org/10.1016/j.ctcp.2014.07.002.

63 "Can Massage Relieve Symptoms of Depression, Anxiety and Stress?" Mayo Clinic, July 20, 2033, https://www.mayoclinichealthsystem.org/hometown-health/speaking-of-health/massage-for-depression-anxiety-and-stress.

64 Maria Meier et al., "Standardized Massage Interventions as Protocols for the Induction of Psychophysiological Relaxation in the Laboratory: A Block Randomized, Controlled Trial," *Scientific Reports* 10, no. 1 (September 8, 2020), https://doi.org/10.1038/s41598-020-71173-w.

65 Wan-An Lu, Gau-Yang Chen, and Cheng-Deng Kuo, "Foot Reflexology Can Increase Vagal Modulation, Decrease Sympathetic Modulation, and Lower Blood Pressure in Healthy Subjects and Patients with Coronary Artery Disease," *Alternative Therapies in Health and Medicine* 17, no. 4 (July-August 2011): 8–14, https://pubmed.ncbi.nlm.nih.gov/22314629/.

66 Malin Henriksson et al., "Effects of Exercise on Symptoms of Anxiety in Primary Care Patients: A Randomized Controlled Trial," *Journal of Affective Disorders* 15, no. 297 (February 2022): 26–34, https://doi.org/10.1016/j.jad.2021.10.006.

67 Habib, *Activate Your Vagus Nerve*, 155–156.

68 "Physical Activity Guidelines for Americans," 2nd ed, US Department of Health and Human Services, June 2023, https://health.gov/sites/default/files/2019-09/Physical_Activity_Guidelines_2nd_edition.pdf.

69 Tina Mäkineni et al., "Autonomic Nervous Function During Whole-Body Cold Exposure Before and After Cold Acclimation," *Aviation, Space, and*

Environmental Medicine (September 2008): 26, 34, https://doi.org/10.3357/asem.2235.2008.

70 "Why Cold Water Is Dangerous," National Center for Cold Water Safety, 2023, https://www.coldwatersafety.org/the-danger.

71 Manuela Jungmass, PhD, et al., "Effects of Cold Stimulation on Cardiac-Vagal Activation in Healthy Participants: Randomized Controlled Trial," *Journal of Medical Internet Research* 2, no. 2, (October 9, 2018), https://doi.org/10.2196/10257.

72 Chen-Te Chiang et al., "The Effect of Ice Water Ingestion on Autonomic Modulation in Healthy Subjects," *Clinical Autonomic Research* 20, no. 6 (December 20, 2010): 375–380, https://doi.org/10.1007/s10286-010-0077-3.

73 Yana Hoffman, RD, CCDC, and Hank Davis, PhD, "Sing in the Shower to Make Friends with Your Vagus Nerve," *Psychology Today* (blog), March 17, 2020, https://www.psychologytoday.com/us/blog/try-see-it-my-way/202003/sing-in-the-shower-make-friends-your-vagus-nerve.

74 David A. Camlin et al., "Group Singing as a Resource for the Development of a Healthy Public: A Study of Adult Group Singing," *Humanities and Social Sciences Communications*, 7, no. 60 (August 5, 2020), https://doi.org/10.1057/s41599-020-00549-0.

75 Bangalore G. Kalyani et al., "Neurohemodynamic Correlates of 'OM' Chanting: A Pilot Functional Magnetic Resonance Imaging Study," *International Journal of Yoga* 4, no. 1 (January 2011): 3–6, https://doi.org/10.4103/0973-6131.78171.

76 Cyrus Darki et al., "The Effect of Classical Music on Heart Rate, Blood Pressure, and Mood," *Cureus Journal of Medical Science* 14, no. 7 (July 2022): https://doi.org/10.7759/cureus.27348.

77 Habib, *Activate Your Vagus Nerve*, 150.

78 Ramon Mora-Ripoll, "Simulated Laughter Techniques for Therapeutic Use in Mental Health," *Journal of Psychology and Clinical Psychiatry* 8, no. 2 (October 19, 2017): https://doi.org/10.15406/jpcpy.2017.08.00479.

Acknowledgments

There are some wonderful people who helped make this book possible, and I'm deeply grateful to them all.

I would especially like to thank my husband, Thomas F. Leeds for his love, his support, and his great illustrations. Thanks for making all my dreams come true.

I would also like to thank Grant Leeds, Molly Leeds, Tyler Leeds, Lisa Leeds, and Marilyn Gfroerer for always being there for me.

I would like to thank my amazing friends and support team, Peg Doyle, Lucille Fisher, Martha Henry-Macdonald, and Linda DeRensis. You're the best.

I would also like to thank my fellow writers, Pat Barletta, Linda Grochowalski and Wendy Rogalinski. You're the best.

I feel so lucky to get to work with two amazing professionals, Michael Boezi, and Sharon Tousley. Thanks for always going the extra mile and making it look like I know what I'm doing.

Thanks to my incredible, talented editors Lindsey Alexander and Sal Borriello, to my copyeditor, Laura Major, and to my designer, Liz Schreiter. It's a joy to work with you and your team.

I'm grateful to my wonderful friends, Marilyn Richards, Cheryl Clark, Joanne Crowell, Ruth Dunnavan, Nancy Farwell, Roberta Rosenthal Hawkins, Jeannie Ryder, and Barbie Talbot, And thanks to my gifted professional colleagues, Hollis Burkhart, Michelle Harris, and Sister Jacqueline LeBoeuf. I feel lucky to know you all.

About Wendy Leeds

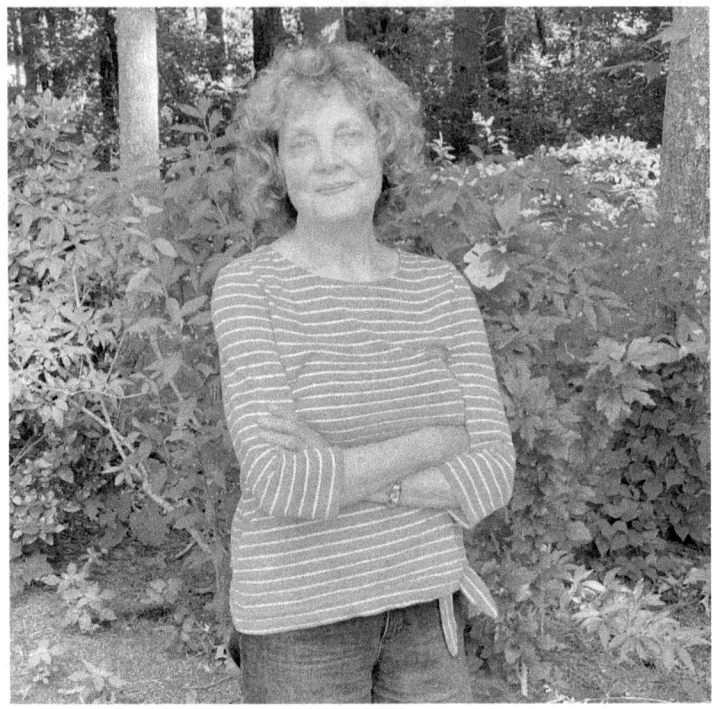

As a three-time cancer survivor, Wendy Leeds is an expert on what it's like to live with anxiety.

As an experienced, licensed psychotherapist, Wendy's mission is to help anxious people everywhere learn to acknowledge and ease their anxiety.

Her work empowers people to create the calm-centered lives they deserve.

Wendy lives in Massachusetts with her husband, Tom, and their dog, Myles Standish.

More about Wendy: wendyleeds.com/about
Connect with Wendy: wendyleeds.com/links

www.ingramcontent.com/pod-product-compliance
Lightning Source LLC
LaVergne TN
LVHW011826060526
838200LV00053B/3909